Training Techniques in Cardiac Rehabilitation

Current Issues in Cardiac Rehabilitation Series

Monograph Number 3

Paul S. Fardy, PhD, Queens College, Flushing, New York,
CICR Series Editor;
Barry A. Franklin, PhD,
William Beaumont Hospital, Royal Oak, Michigan;
John P. Porcari, PhD,
University of Wisconsin, LaCrosse, Wisconsin;
David E. Verrill, MS,
Mid-Carolina Cardiology, Charlotte, North Carolina

Human Kinetics Publishers

Library of Congress Cataloguing-in-Publication Data

Training techniques in cardiac rehabilitation /
   Paul S. Fardy . . . [et al.].
       p. cm. -- (Current issues in cardiac rehabilitation, ISSN
   1071-7889 ; monograph no. 3)
       Includes bibliographical references and index.
       ISBN 0-87322-536-8
       1. Heart--Diseases--Exercise therapy. 2. Heart--Diseases-
   -Patients--Rehabilitation. 3. Patient education. I. Fardy, Paul
   S. II. Series.
       [DNLM: 1. Coronary Disease--rehabilitation. 2. Exercise.
   3. Patient Care Planning. W1 CU788KQ no. 3 1998 / WG 300 T768 1998]
   RC684.E9T73 1998.
   616.1'2062--dc21
   DNLM/DLC
   for Library of Congress   97-16033
                                                                           CIP

ISBN: 0-87322-536-8
ISSN: 1071-7889

Developmental Editor: Elaine Mustain; **Assistant Editor:** Sarah Wiseman, Sandra Merz Bott, Melinda Graham; **Editorial Assistants:** Amy Carnes, Laura Majersky, Ted Sammons; **Copyeditor:** Joyce Sexton; **Proofreader:** Tom Long; **Indexer:** Craig Brown; **Graphic Designer:** Keith Blomberg; **Graphic Artist:** Roberta R. Edwards; **Photo Editor:** Boyd LaFoon; **Cover Designer:** Keith Blomberg; **Photographer (interior):** chapter 2-Ervin Jackson and Jim Simpson; chapter 3-John Zoerb; **Illustrator:** Patricia Banks; **Printer:** United Graphics

Printed in the United States of America   10 9 8 7 6 5 4 3 2 1

Human Kinetics Publishers
Web site: http://www.humankinetics.com/

United States: Human Kinetics
Box 5076, Champaign, IL 61825-5076
1-800-747-4457
e-mail: humank@hkusa.com

Canada: Human Kinetics, Box 24040, Windsor, ON N8Y 4Y9
1-800-465-7301 (in Canada only)
e-mail: humank@hkcanada.com

Europe: Human Kinetics
P.O. Box 1W14, Leeds LS16 6TR, United Kingdom
(44) 1132 781708
e-mail: humank@hkeurope.com

Australia: Human Kinetics, 57A Price Avenue, Lower Mitcham, South Australia 5062
(08) 277 1555
e-mail: humank@hkaustralia.com

New Zealand: Human Kinetics, P.O. Box 105-231, Auckland 1
(09) 523 3462
e-mail: humank@hknewz.com

Contents

Preface

The science of prescribing exercise for cardiac patients has progressed over the years, and cardiac patients today can expect a far different exercise prescription and training regimen than patients 20 years ago. Many studies have demonstrated efficacy and safety from a widely expanded armamentarium of exercises and training techniques. Patient numbers have also expanded as a result of greater numbers of programs, liberalization of eligibility criteria, and risk stratification that have opened the door for greater at-home participation. Exercise programs for cardiac patients have become increasingly sophisticated, comprehensive, and diversified, enabling more patients to participate with increased safety and benefit and with a greater likelihood of long-term adherence.

Nevertheless, data on long-term adherence remain rather discouraging, regardless of the type of intervention. Many more controlled studies are needed to identify adherers and nonadherers, especially investigations of psychological characteristics. Program delivery strategies must also be assessed critically to determine their influence on adherence and compliance. Two things are clear, however: that having fun and feeling better are important determinants of adherence, and that in the final analysis our efforts are of little value if the patients we treat don't make a lifetime commitment to a healthier lifestyle.

As the scope of cardiac rehabilitation programs continues to increase and a greater variety of patients with increased disease are included, it becomes more clear that exercise prescription and training is an art as well as a science—that the professional staff are often in the position of using their best guess based on accepted scientific rationale. Therefore, the primary goal of *Training Techniques in Cardiac Rehabilitation* is to offer the program director and exercise leader in-depth information on nontraditional programs currently available to the practitioner, providing tools to enhance both the art and science of our decision making.

The monograph starts with a chapter describing the latest research on general principles of exercise prescription, including findings on how various medications affect patients' abilities to exercise. The next three chapters deal with the specifics of resistance training, aquatics programming, and flexibility and aerobic training through group ball games. Each of the latter three chapters contains not only principles of prescription but also practical program information, to an increasing extent. Because most practitioners are already familiar with weight training, and because the options for resistance training are so numerous, the chapter on resistance training does not present much information on specific exercises but rather guides the practitioner through the process of writing programs using appropriate exercises for specific patients. The aquatics chapter provides extensive information on safety as well as on principles of aquatic exercise prescription, closing with a discussion of aquatic exercises including water aerobics, swimming, and water volleyball. Because games programming is a relatively new option, the bulk of the final chapter is devoted to specific games that may be used in your rehabilitation program, including information on the rehabilitative benefits of each activity. The authors provide background literature and draw on vast personal experience in program implementation and benefits.

It is hoped and expected that this monograph will be of value as you plan and develop new programs, provide increased options while maintaining safety and efficacy, and rethink the goals and procedures of existing options. Our intention is to provide you with a variety of alternatives as well as an understanding of how, when, where, and why they are used. We hope that you will find this material interesting and useful.

The Authors

Acknowledgments

Thank you to my assistants Ann Azzolini and Shayne Kohn for running our program so well and enabling me to do these other things.   *—Paul Fardy*

Thank you to Dee LaPointe for her assistance and tireless efforts in the meticulous preparation of these manuscripts.   *—Barry A. Franklin*

Thank you to John Zoerb for his help in taking the photos that appear in my chapter.   *—John Porcari*

Thank you to my wife, Susie, for the time, dedication, and devotion she has given me during the writing of this chapter. Thanks also to the members of the North Carolina Cardiopulmonary Rehabilitation Association for their support, suggestions, and implementation of cardiac resistive exercise training in their programs.   *—David E. Verrill*

Chapter 1

Exercise Evaluation, Prescription, and Training

Barry A. Franklin, PhD

Paul S. Fardy, PhD

P rescribing exercise for cardiac patients is both a science and an art. It is comparable in many ways to prescribing medications; that is, one recommends an optimal dosage according to individual needs and limitations. In the case of exercise dosage, or training stimulus, the prescription consists of an intensity, a duration, a frequency, and a mode of activity. These should be periodically adjusted to maximize safety and promote optimal improvement.

The scientific basis of the exercise prescription is well established for most cardiac patients (1). For some patients, however, limited data are available and the prescription is more an art than a science. Examples of patients for whom the scientific knowledge base is incomplete are those with extremely low physical work capacity complicated by symptoms, those with heart failure, the very elderly, and cardiac transplant recipients, in whom myriad physical and psychological factors need to be considered.

The purpose of this chapter is to review the physiologic basis and rationale for exercise therapy in patients who have heart disease, with specific reference to patient eligibility, the preliminary evaluation, exercise prescription, concomitant drug therapy, safety, chronic adaptations to training, and issues regarding motivation and compliance.

Patient Eligibility

Many reports and position papers reflect the consensus of national medical organizations that exercise-based cardiac rehabilitation has become the "standard of care" within the medical community by which a broad spectrum of patients are restored to their optimal physical, medical, and psychosocial status after an acute cardiac event (2). This includes the traditional patients of past years—myocardial infarction, coronary bypass, and angioplasty patients—in addition to the following: coronary patients with or without residual myocardial ischemia, left ventricular dysfunction, and arrhythmias; a variety of categories of patients with nonischemic heart disease; patients with concomitant pulmonary disease; patients who have undergone pacemaker or cardioverter-defibrillator implantation, heart valve repair or replacement, and cardiac transplantation; elderly patients; patients with additional medical disorders such as hypertension, peripheral vascular disease, and diabetes mellitus; and medically complex patients taking multiple medications. Virtually all of these patient subsets have demonstrated improved exercise tolerance as a result of comprehensive rehabilitation programs.

Absolute Contraindications

There are, however, absolute contraindications that may preclude some patients from participating in the exercise component of the rehabilitation program. These include unstable angina pectoris, selected structural cardiac abnormalities, severe coronary artery disease (CAD), serious ventricular arrhythmias or rhythm disturbances, and other medical conditions that could be aggravated by exercise (1). Although these patients are still candidates for education and counseling, they may require medical and/or surgical interventions before initiating the exercise component.

Questionable Cases

Recently, questions have arisen about the advisability of vigorous exercise training for two patient subsets: those with exertional ST-segment depression ($\geq$1 mm) without symptoms and those recovering from myocardial infarction involving a large portion of the anterior wall (3). Some clinicians have suggested that the former should refrain from vigorous exercise training, citing biopsy studies of ischemic myocardium showing increased fibrosis (4). Silent myocardial ischemia may also increase the risk of cardiac arrest during vigorous physical exertion (5). One widely publicized report suggested that some patients may respond adversely to exercise training soon after large anterior wall myocardial infarction, demonstrating further deterioration in global and regional left ventricular function as compared to nonexercising control patients (6). However, other investigations of silent ischemia have allayed concerns regarding risk, demonstrating better survival, milder disease, and higher exercise-training intensities in such patients as compared to those with symptoms (7-9). In addition, two recent randomized controlled trials (10, 11) in patients with anterior Q-wave myocardial infarction and decreased ejection fraction indicate that infarct expansion and a further deterioration in left ventricular function are unlikely outcomes of exercise training.

Evaluation

An individualized and comprehensive exercise prescription requires a thorough patient evaluation, as outlined in table 1.1 (12). Background data may be collected from physical measurements, questionnaires, and personal interviews. The latter generally have greater validity, provide more detailed information, and allow for follow-up questions, but require more time to administer.

Table 1.1   Patient Evaluation

1. Physical measurements	Height, weight, body mass index, percent body fat, systolic and diastolic blood pressure, lipid profile, waist and hip girth
2. Lifestyle history	Cigarette smoking, diet, and physical activity habits
3. Medical history	Personal and immediate family history of cardiovascular disease including major coronary risk factors
4. Physical limitations	Any neurologic, vascular, or orthopedic impairment that would limit exercise
5. Activity preference	Leisure activities that are of interest for long-term programming
6. Exercise tolerance	Preferably a sign/symptom–limited exercise test on one or more test modes that are specific to training goals
7. Goals and objectives	A list of short- and long-range goals

Physical measurements such as height, weight, body mass index, percent body fat, hip and waist circumference, blood pressure, and lipid/lipoprotein profile provide a basis for future comparison and identify major coronary risk factors. *Lifestyle habits and medical history* should also be obtained to develop health promotion programs that complement the exercise-training program. *Physical limitations* that may affect the exercise prescription should be identified in the preliminary medical history. Musculoskeletal assessment by a physical therapist may be helpful in this regard, especially for elderly patients and those with a history of neurologic, vascular, or orthopedic impairment of the lower extremities.

The patient's *preference for physical activity* is especially useful in planning an exercise-training program. Long-term adherence will be more likely to occur when the patient perceives exercise as enjoyable and beneficial. In some instances, one may have to modify activities or provide alternatives to activities that the patient dislikes. Personal preference, however, should not preclude the introduction of new activities by the program staff.

Measuring *exercise tolerance* and, if possible, aerobic capacity, is an important part of the evaluation in developing the activity prescription. Results from the exercise test help establish safe intensities for training the lower and/or upper extremities (13) and identify occupational and leisure-time activities that are appropriate for the patient's physical work capacity.

Functional Exercise Testing

The most widely recognized measure of cardiopulmonary fitness is the aerobic capacity or maximal oxygen consumption ($\dot{V}O_2max$). This variable is defined physiologically as the highest rate of oxygen transport and use that can be achieved at maximal physical exertion. Because true $\dot{V}O_2max$ in cardiac patients is seldom achieved due to abnormal signs, symptoms, or volitional fatigue, this variable is often termed $\dot{V}O_2$ peak in this population.

Somatic oxygen consumption ($\dot{V}O_2$) may be expressed mathematically by a rearrangement of the Fick equation: $\dot{V}O_2 = HR \times SV \times (CaO_2 - C\bar{v}O_2)$, where $\dot{V}O_2$ is oxygen consumption in milliliters per minute, HR is heart rate in beats per minute, SV is stroke volume in milliliters per beat, and $CaO_2 - C\bar{v}O_2$ is the arteriovenous oxygen difference in milliliters of oxygen per deciliter of blood. Accordingly, both central and peripheral regulatory mechanisms affect the magnitude of body oxygen consumption.

Expression of $\dot{V}O_2$max

Maximal oxygen consumption may be expressed on an absolute basis in liters per minute, reflecting total body energy output and caloric expenditure, where each liter of oxygen consumed is equivalent to approximately 5 kilocalories. Because large persons usually have a large absolute oxygen consumption simply by virtue of their large muscle mass, physiologists generally divide this value by body weight in kilograms to allow a more equitable comparison among individuals of different size. This variable, when expressed in milliliters of oxygen per kilogram of body weight per minute (ml · kg · min^{-1}) or as metabolic equivalents (METs; 1 MET = approximately 3.5 ml · kg · min), is considered the single best index of physical work capacity or cardiopulmonary fitness (14).

Determination of $\dot{V}O_2$max

Maximal oxygen consumption ($\dot{V}O_2$max) is generally determined by measuring the volume and analyzing the oxygen and carbon dioxide content of the subject's expired air during the last minutes of an exercise test. Traditionally, this variable has been measured using an open-circuit or Douglas bag technique. However, numerous automated metabolic measurement systems have now become available.

Because direct measurement of oxygen consumption is sometimes inconvenient, requiring sophisticated equipment, technical expertise, and frequent calibration, clinicians have increasingly sought to predict or estimate $\dot{V}O_2$max from the treadmill speed and percent grade (see figs. 1.1 and 1.2), or the cycle ergometer work rate, expressed as kilogram meters per minute. It is important to remember, however, that the cardiac patient's peak oxygen uptake may be markedly overestimated when it is predicted from exercise time or workload (15).

Several explanations have been offered to clarify the discrepancy between measured and predicted $\dot{V}O_2$ values in cardiac patients. Previously published aerobic requirements for progressive work rates were generally derived from healthy young adults, and they apply only when the subject has achieved steady state conditions without holding the treadmill handrails. It has also been suggested that left ventricular dysfunction and beta-adrenergic blocking medications may slow oxygen uptake kinetics, resulting in lower submaximal and peak oxygen uptake values for standard work rates (16, 17).

Postevaluation Consult

The professional staff, program participant, and significant others should meet after the initial evaluation to clarify what the patient hopes to accomplish, that is, to establish short- and long-range goals and objectives (12). Because achieving one's goals is a powerful motivator, the goals should be clear to those persons comprising the patient's sup-

METs	1.6	2	3	4	5	6	7	8	9	10	11	12	13	14	15	16
Balke							3.4 miles/hr									
				2	4	6	8	10	12	14	16	18	20	22	24	26
Balke						3.0 miles/hr										
			0	2.5	5	7.5	10	12.5	15	17.5	20	22.5				
Naughton	1.0		2.0 miles/hr													
	0	0	3.5	7	10.5	14	17.5									
METs	1.6	2	3	4	5	6	7	8	9	10	11	12	13	14	15	16
O$_2$,ml/kg/min	5.6	7		14		21		28		35		42		49		56
Clinical status	Symptomatic patients															
	Diseased, recovered															
			Sedentary healthy													
				Physically active subjects												
Functional class	IV		III			II		I and normal								

Figure 1.1 Metabolic cost of selected treadmill test protocols. A MET is a unit of energy expenditure equivalent to approximately 3.5 milliliters of oxygen uptake per kilogram of body weight per minute (ml/kg/min). Numbers refer to treadmill speed (top) and percentage grade (bottom).

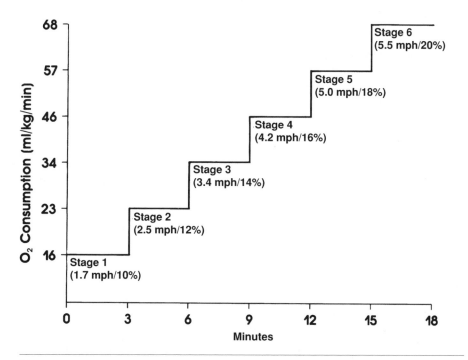

Figure 1.2 The standard Bruce treadmill protocol showing progressive stages (speed, percentage grade) and the corresponding aerobic requirements, expressed as ml/kg/min.

port system. The professional staff evaluates whether the patient's goals are realistic and outlines steps for their achievement. Specific objectives of the meeting should include

1. identifying exercise preferences;
2. identifying a realistic sequence of short- and long-range goals;
3. providing the patient and significant family members or friends with an opportunity to meet the staff;
4. allaying anxiety and apprehension;
5. having the patient, family, and friends view the equipment and facilities;
6. having the patient, family, and friends ask questions about the program; and
7. making sure that everyone is familiar with the goals of the patient.

This meeting provides an excellent opportunity for the professional staff to clarify the benefits of cardiac rehabilitation to the patient and his/her significant others. Because of psychological trauma, medications, and a host of potential distractions following an acute cardiac event, the goal-setting session may be one of the first opportunities for the patient to assess the value of lifestyle changes. The goal-setting meeting should be well thought out, meaningful, and informative, and should be an integral part of the total cardiac rehabilitation program. It is also an opportunity for the professional staff to learn about the patient's lifestyle—information that can be helpful in assessing goals—and to outline the exercise prescription and complementary risk reduction programs.

Exercise Prescription

When it comes to the benefits of regular exercise, increased cardiorespiratory fitness is often emphasized more than the potential for improved health and disease prevention. There are, however, many health benefits of moderate exercise intensities, including favorable changes in bone density, improved glucose tolerance, and improved coronary risk factors, as well as a reduction in cardiovascular-related mortality.

Figure 1.3 shows the theoretical relationship between health and fitness benefits expected from increasing doses of exercise (12, 18). Gains in aerobic fitness are modest until the intensity approximates 50-60% $\dot{V}O_2$max, at which time improvement is rapid; a plateauing then occurs between 85% and 90% of functional capacity. It is apparent that health benefits can occur at lower intensities of exercise (e.g., less than 50% $\dot{V}O_2$max) than are generally prescribed for cardiorespiratory conditioning. Such programs, however, are usually associated with longer and/or more frequent exercise sessions.

Intensity

The prescribed exercise intensity should be above a minimal level required to induce a "training effect," yet below the metabolic rate that evokes abnormal clinical signs or symptoms (e.g., ischemic ST-segment depression, angina pectoris, threatening ventricular arrhythmias). For most deconditioned cardiac patients, the threshold intensity for exercise training probably lies between 40% and 60% $\dot{V}O_2$max (19); however, consider-

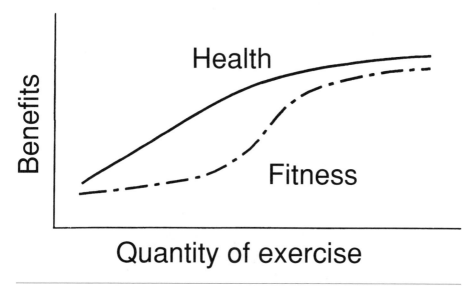

Figure 1.3   Theoretical relation between health and fitness benefits and the amount or intensity of exercise.

able evidence suggests that it increases in direct proportion to the pretraining $\dot{V}O_2max$ or level of habitual physical activity (see fig. 1.4). Improvement in aerobic capacity with low to moderate training intensities suggests that the interrelation among the training intensity, frequency, and duration may permit a decrease in the intensity to be partially or totally compensated for by increases in the exercise duration or frequency, or both.

Establishing the Target Heart Rate

To attain a desired metabolic load for exercise training, one must either measure the oxygen uptake directly or have an equivalent index thereof. The strong linear relationship between oxygen uptake and heart rate during dynamic exercise involving large muscle groups provides the basis for the exercise prescription (12). Consequently, a predetermined training or target heart rate range has become widely adopted as an indicator of exercise intensity (20).

Training heart rates for cardiorespiratory conditioning are commonly determined by one of three methods from data obtained during graded treadmill or cycle ergometer testing: (a) the heart rate versus oxygen uptake regression method, (b) the percentage of maximal (peak) heart rate method, and (c) the Karvonen or heart rate reserve method.

The first method involves identifying the heart rate that occurred at a given oxygen uptake or MET level during a progressive exercise test either to volitional fatigue or to a sign- or symptom-limited endpoint (21). The target heart rate range is equal to the heart rate (± 6 beats/min) that occurred at a given oxygen uptake or MET load (e.g., 50-80% of aerobic capacity). This method is most accurate when steady-state heart rate and oxygen uptake are determined during several progressive submaximal work rates.

The second method widely used to compute the target heart rate is to calculate a fixed percentage (e.g., 70-85%) of the measured maximal heart rate (22). This method

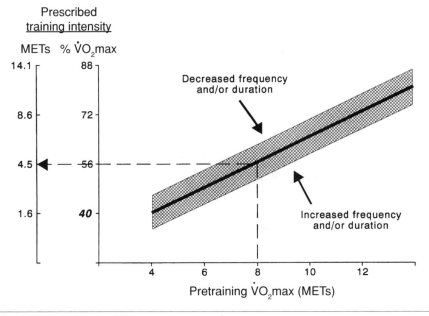

Figure 1.4　Theoretical relation between aerobic capacity (METs) and the minimal intensity for exercise training, expressed as a percentage of the maximal oxygen uptake ($\dot{V}O_2$max). The threshold intensity for training increases in direct proportion to $\dot{V}O_2$max before training; however, it can be modulated by altering the exercise duration or frequency, or both. For example, a patient with an aerobic capacity of 8 METs would exercise at approximately 56% of his/her $\dot{V}O_2$max, or 4.5 ± 0.5 METs, to further increase his/her functional capacity.

has been shown to yield similar regressions of percentage $\dot{V}O_2$max on percentage HRmax (i.e., 60-80% $\dot{V}O_2$max is approximately equal to 70-85% HRmax) regardless of gender, the presence or absence of CAD, aerobic fitness, body weight and fat stores, muscle groups involved, exercise testing mode, or cardiac medications (23, 24). However, limitations of the method include the underestimation of the target heart rate for a given MET level (1) and considerable individual variability in the relationship between relative heart rate and oxygen uptake when these are expressed as percentages of their respective maximum values (25).

The final method of establishing the target heart rate is the maximal heart rate reserve method of Karvonen et al. (26), in which the training heart rate = (maximal heart rate – resting heart rate) × 50-80%, plus resting heart rate. This method, which requires reliable measurements of resting (standing) and maximal heart rate, closely approximates measuring the percentage of aerobic capacity in healthy young men (27). However, it may overestimate the desired aerobic training intensity in cardiac patients, particularly during the early stages of rehabilitation (28).

A comparison of the second and third prescriptive methods, using a standardized training intensity (i.e., 70%) with varied resting heart rates, is shown in table 1.2. The Karvonen formula calculates the training intensity as a percentage of the heart rate reserve rather than as a fixed percentage of the maximal heart rate. The straight percentage method yielded the lowest training heart rate. In contrast, target heart rates for the Karvonen method increased as a function of the resting heart rate.

The MET Method of Exercise Prescription

Another acceptable method of prescribing exercise intensity is by metabolic equivalents, or METs, which represent multiples of the resting metabolic rate. One MET is equivalent to the metabolic rate at rest, or approximately 3.5 ml O_2/kg/min. Two METs, therefore, equals twice the resting metabolic rate (i.e., 7.0 ml/kg/min), and so on. Prescribing exercise by METs uses whole numbers that are assigned to physical activities. The prescription represents a percentage of peak METs achieved on the exercise test. For example, if 10 METs are attained on an exercise test and the training intensity is set at 70%, then activities of 7 METs or slightly less are appropriate. Published values of the aerobic requirements of common occupational and recreational activities are available elsewhere (29).

The MET method is easier and less intrusive for the patient than palpating the pulse and counting heart rates. However, common errors include the following:

- **Using published values as precise measurements.** METs represent only an estimate of energy expenditure unless resting and exercise oxygen uptake are directly measured. Because resting metabolic rate varies among individuals and is influenced by factors such as physical condition, body size, and medications (30), actual METs may also vary from published values. Therefore, tables of metabolic equivalents represent only average values and should be used conservatively.
- **Failure to allow for effects of skill and competition.** Activities that require a high level of skill have widely varying MET values, whereas activities with minimal skill, such as walking, jogging, and bicycling, have considerably less variability (29). Competition can also increase the MET cost of any given recreational activity.
- **Assuming that somatic oxygen consumption always provides an accurate estimate of cardiac demand.** One cannot assume that all occupational work demanding

Table 1.2   Comparison of Target Heart Rates Calculated by the Fixed Percentage and Karvonen Methods Using Varied Resting Heart Rates

Method	% of maximal heart rate	Karvonen formula	
Maximal heart rate (beats/min)	150	150	150
Resting heart rate (beats/min)	—	50	80
Training intensity (%)	70	70	70
Target heart rate (beats/min)	105	120	129

oxygen consumption equal to that registered during leg exercise testing produces similar heart rate and systolic blood pressure responses (myocardial oxygen demand). Additional factors at work include the stresses of emotions, excitement, cognition, temperature (see fig. 1.5) (31), and humidity, as well as the activation of muscle groups not used during the exercise tests.

- **Incorrectly determining METs during the exercise test.** Previously published aerobic requirements for individual work rates of an exercise test assume steady state conditions and are population specific. Moreover, the MET cost of treadmill walking is relatively constant, regardless of body weight, whereas the relative aerobic requirements of cycle ergometry are weight dependent. Thus, a given work rate on the treadmill (e.g., 3.0 miles/hour, 0% grade) requires approximately the same relative oxygen consumption, 3 METs or 10.5 ml/kg/min, for all persons, whereas the MET cost of a given power output on the cycle ergometer varies inversely with body weight.

- **Underestimating a patient's physical work capacity.** Estimated oxygen costs are commonly derived from continuous steady state work (≥ 3 min), whereas many activities of daily life are intermittent rather than continuous. Accordingly, a cardiac patient with a 5 MET capacity might be advised to avoid gardening (a requirement of 5-7 METs), since presumably it represents maximal or supramaximal effort. However, if the activity is performed intermittently (i.e., 1.5 min work, 1.5 min rest), the task can be easily accomplished at oxygen consumption levels well below those estimated for continuous work (32).

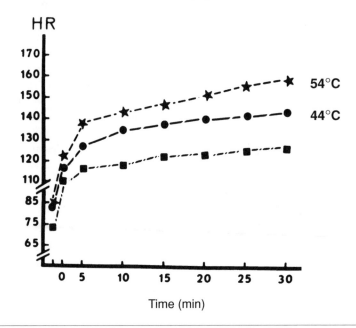

Figure 1.5   Influence of environmental temperature on heart rate responses at a constant work rate over time. Heart rate (HR) increases approximately 1 beat/min for each degree Celsius increment in ambient temperature above 24 °C. Adapted from Pandolf et al. (31).

Because of these potential errors, it may be preferable to prescribe exercise using more precise physiologic data (e.g., heart rate), especially when cardiac demands are critical. Previous studies (33, 34) have shown a good correlation between measured myocardial oxygen consumption and the heart rate response to exercise ($r = 0.88$). On the other hand, METs or perceived exertion may provide a more accurate index of exercise intensity in patients with pacemakers or in cardiac transplant recipients (35, 36).

Rating of Perceived Exertion

The rating of perceived exertion (RPE) is a useful and important adjunct to heart rate as an intensity guide for exercise training. The category and category-ratio scales consist of 15 grades from 6 to 20 and 10 grades from 0 to 10^+ (see fig. 1.6), respectively (37). The ratings, based on one's overall feeling of exertion and physical fatigue, correlate highly

Perceived Exertion

Category scale

6	
7	Very, very light
8	
9	Very light
10	
11	Fairly light
12	
13	Somewhat hard
14	
15	Hard
16	
17	Very hard
18	
19	Very, very hard
20	

Category-ratio scale

0	Nothing at all	
0.5	Very, very weak	[just noticeable]
1	Very weak	
2	Weak	[light]
3	Moderate	
4	Somewhat strong	
5	Strong	[heavy]
6		
7	Very strong	
8		
9		
10	Very, very strong	[almost max]

Maximal

Figure 1.6   Perceived exertion scales with descriptive "effort ratings."

with metabolic responses to exercise (e.g., heart rate, oxygen consumption), particularly when these variables are expressed as percentages of their respective maximums. Participants are advised not to overemphasize any one sensation, such as leg pain or dyspnea, but to try to assess their total, inner feelings of exertion. However, clinical experience suggests that a small percentage of participants (~10%) tend to select unrealistic or invalid RPE scores despite standardized instructions (1). Among healthy young persons, the effort rating on the category scale generally approximates 1/10 of the heart rate response.

Exercise rated as 11 to 13 (6-20 scale) or 3 to 4 (0-10 scale), between "fairly light" and "somewhat hard" (6-20 scale) or between "moderate" and "somewhat strong" (0-10 scale)—corresponding to 60-70% of the maximal heart rate (or 45-60% $\dot{V}O_2$max)—generally yields health-related benefits. In contrast, exercise rated 13 to 16 (6-20 scale), between "somewhat hard" and "hard," or 4 to 6 (0-10 scale), between "somewhat strong and very strong"—corresponding to 70-85% of maximal heart rate (or 60-80% $\dot{V}O_2$max)—is generally considered more appropriate for cardiorespiratory conditioning.

The concept of perceived exertion appears to be valid even for patients whose heart rates are attenuated by propranolol, since similar RPEs are obtained at a given percentage of maximum heart rate reserve regardless of the beta blocker dosage or peak heart rate (38). However, there are limitations in using RPE alone to gauge exercise intensity. Although the subjective rating correlates well with heart rate, oxygen uptake, and workload, ischemic ST-segment depression and threatening ventricular dysrhythmias can occur without symptoms at low RPEs (39).

Frequency

Although exercise is usually prescribed for 3 or 4 days per week, recent studies suggest that two exercise sessions per week are as effective as three per week for cardiorespiratory conditioning in the early weeks of phase II cardiac rehabilitation (40). The training regimens of two and three sessions per week produced similar increases in treadmill time and aerobic capacity and decreases in submaximal heart rate (see fig. 1.7). Studies in healthy middle-aged men suggest that the additional aerobic benefits of five training sessions per week appear to be minimal, whereas the incidence of lower-extremity injuries increases abruptly (41).

Duration

The duration of exercise required to elicit a significant training effect varies inversely with the intensity; the greater the intensity (up to about 80% $\dot{V}O_2$max), the shorter the duration of exercise necessary to achieve favorable adaptation and improvement in cardiorespiratory fitness. Thus, low-intensity exercise may be partially or totally compensated for by a longer exercise duration. Exercise training for 5-10 minutes improves aerobic capacity (42), and 30-minute sessions are even more effective (43). However, longer training sessions (≥45 min) are associated with a disproportionate incidence of orthopedic injury (41).

Recently, investigators studied healthy middle-aged men who completed three 10-minute bouts of moderate-intensity exercise per day versus those who performed one

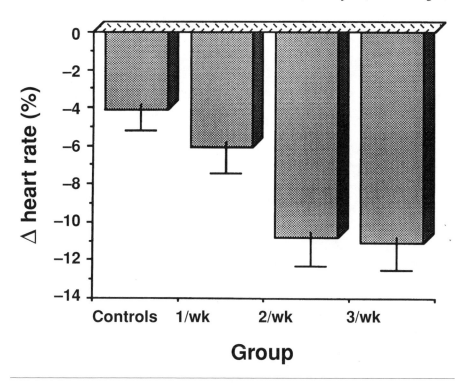

Figure 1.7   Percentage decreases (mean ± SE) in submaximal heart rate after an exercise-based cardiac rehabilitation program. From Dressendorfer et al. (40).

"long" exercise bout of 30 minutes, 5 days per week for 8 weeks (44). Although the relative increase in measured maximal oxygen consumption was significantly greater in the long-bout group (13.9% vs. 7.6%), the two groups demonstrated identical percentage increases and decreases in exercise test duration and submaximal heart rate, respectively (see table 1.3). These findings suggest that multiple short bouts of moderate-intensity physical exercise produce significant training effects. For some patients, this exercise regimen may fit better into a busy schedule than a single long bout.

Progressing the Prescription

Some training adaptation usually occurs within 6 weeks, although the rate of improvement is highly individualized (12). As the heart rate response at a fixed level of exertion is reduced, work rates must be increased to achieve the target rate. Thus, initial changes in the exercise prescription concentrate on increasing physical work. After the work rate has been increased one or more times, the training target heart rate may also be increased to a slightly higher percentage of maximum (e.g., from 70% to 75%). A 5% increase is common, although the specific recommendation is based on individual patient improvement, age, and clinical status. Training adaptation is more rapid early in the physical conditioning program as compared with the rate of improvement later on.

Table 1.3   Training Effects of Long Versus Short Bouts of Exercise in Healthy Subjects*

Variable/program	Long (30 min) (% Δ)	Short (3-10 min) (% Δ)
$\dot{V}O_2$max (ml/kg/min)	+13.9[a]	+7.6
Treadmill time (min)	+12	+12
Submaximal exercise heart rate	−6	−6

[a]$p = 0.03$ versus short bouts; %Δ = percentage change.
*DeBusk et al. (44).

Training Techniques and Modalities

Exercise training has undergone evolutionary changes in objectives and content since the early days of cardiac rehabilitation. Twenty years ago, exercise-based cardiac rehabilitation programs consisted largely of continuous walking and stationary cycle ergometry. It was widely believed that continuous aerobic exercise of large muscles in the lower body was the only safe type of training for cardiac patients. Considerably less information was available about other modes of exercise. Upper-body exercise in particular was believed to cause increased arrhythmias and myocardial ischemia, and was generally prohibited.

Training techniques developed for the National Exercise and Heart Disease Project (45) signaled a significant change in exercise for cardiac patients. For the first time the specificity of exercise, long recognized as an important training principle for athletes, was incorporated into cardiac rehabilitation to encourage a return to specific work tasks and leisure activities. Training techniques in addition to continuous and aerobic exercise were also introduced and were shown to be safe, appropriate, and often advantageous for cardiac patients (46). In particular, intermittent training that utilized muscles of the upper (13) and lower body and a variety of exercise modes was established as safe and beneficial. Currently, most cardiac rehabilitation exercise-training programs include aspects of continuous and intermittent training. Moreover, resistance training has been shown to improve skeletal muscle strength and endurance in clinically stable coronary patients (2).

The physiologic adaptations to exercise training appear to be largely specific to the muscle groups that have been conditioned. Clausen et al. (47) demonstrated that leg training caused a significant reduction in the heart rate response to leg exercise, but not to arm exercise. Conversely, arm training resulted in an attenuated heart rate response to arm exercise, but not to leg exercise (see fig. 1.8). Similar "muscle-specific" adaptations have been shown for blood lactate and pulmonary ventilation (48, 49), suggesting that a significant portion of the training response derives from peripheral rather than central changes, including cellular and enzymatic adaptations that increase the oxidative capacity of chronically exercised skeletal muscle (50).

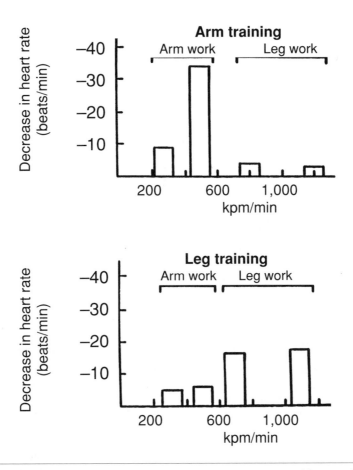

Figure 1.8   The effects of training on the heart rate response to arm and leg exercise. Adapted from Clausen et al. (47).

The lack of transfer of training benefits from one set of limbs to another appears to discredit the general practice of prescribing exercise for the legs alone. Many occupational and leisure-time activities require arm work to a greater extent than leg work (32). Consequently, one should advise cardiac patients who rely on their upper extremities to train the arms as well as the legs, with the expectation of improved cardiorespiratory and hemodynamic responses to both types of effort (13).

Upper-body exercise training for cardiac patients has been traditionally contraindicated, but at a given heart rate, arm exercise elicits no greater incidence of dysrhythmias, ischemic ST-segment depression, or angina pectoris than does leg exercise (51). Moreover, recent studies suggest that the upper extremities respond to aerobic exercise conditioning in the same qualitative and quantitative manner as the lower extremities, showing comparable relative decreases in submaximal rate-pressure product and increases in peak power output and aerobic fitness for both sets of limbs when the same exercise-training intensity, frequency, and duration are used for the arms and legs (52).

Arm Exercise Prescription

Guidelines for arm exercise training should include recommendations regarding three variables (53):

1. The appropriate exercise heart rate
2. The work rate (kg/min or watts) that will elicit a sufficient metabolic load for training
3. The proper training equipment or modalities

Arm exercise training heart rate.   Although the prescribed heart rate for arm training should, ideally, be based on the results of a progressive arm ergometer test, this may not always be feasible. Research indicates that a slightly lower maximal heart rate is generally obtained during arm exercise than during leg exercise testing (54). Consequently, an arm exercise prescription based on a maximal heart rate obtained during leg ergometry may result in an inappropriately high target heart rate for arm training. As a general guideline, we have found that the prescribed heart rate for leg training should be reduced by approximately 10 beats/min for arm training.

Work rates appropriate for arm training.   With regard to prescribing the appropriate work rates for arm training, it is important to emphasize that although maximal physiologic responses are generally greater during leg exercise than during arm exercise, cardiorespiratory responses during arm exercise are higher for any given submaximal work rate. Consequently, a work rate considered appropriate for leg training will generally be too high for arm training. In our experience, work rates approximating 50% of those used for leg training are generally appropriate for arm training (55). Thus, a patient using 100 watts for leg training would employ 50 watts for arm conditioning, with the expectation of comparable heart rates and perceived exertion ratings.

Arm exercise training equipment and modalities.   Specially designed arm or combined arm/leg ergometers are commonly recommended for upper-extremity training. Other equipment used for upper-body training includes rowing machines, weight-training devices, wall pulleys, light dumbbells, ladder-climbing apparatus, and cross-country skiing simulators. Walking or jogging while pumping handheld weights can also be used to facilitate aerobic training of the upper extremities (56).

Resistance Training

Resistance training results in significant improvements in measures of weight-carrying tolerance and in increases in skeletal muscle strength in clinically stable coronary patients when appropriate instruction and prescriptive guidelines are provided (2). Moreover, signs or symptoms of myocardial ischemia, ventricular irritability, and abnormal hemodynamics occur less frequently during resistance testing than during treadmill testing to volitional fatigue. Increased subendocardial perfusion secondary to the elevated diastolic blood pressure that predictably accompanies resistance exercise may contribute to this response (57).

The rationale to support resistance training as an adjunct to an exercise-based cardiac rehabilitation program stems from several lines of evidence (58). Sustained isometric effort is characterized by a pressor response that is proportionate to the relative intensity (percentage of maximal voluntary contraction), duration, and muscle mass involved (59, 60). Consequently, increased muscular strength should result in an attenuated blood pressure response to any given load, since the load now represents a lower percentage of the maximal voluntary contraction.

Although previous studies have reported that resistance-training programs offer little or no benefit to cardiovascular function, these studies generally evaluated the conditioning response with dynamic treadmill or cycle ergometer testing (61). When heart rate and blood pressure responses to a standardized lifting or isometric test before and after a strength-training regimen have been compared, improvement *has* been reported (62). There are also intriguing data to suggest that strength training can increase both treadmill and cycle ergometer endurance time to fatigue without an accompanying increase in aerobic capacity (see table 1.4) (63). Moreover, regular progressive resistance-exercise training may have a favorable effect on resting blood pressure and lipid and lipoprotein levels (64).

Resistance-training guidelines for selected cardiac patients are provided in chapter 2, with specific reference to the appropriate number of sets and repetitions, progression, proper breathing technique, and safety concerns. Interestingly, heavy-resistance exercise, which may potentially increase the hemodynamic response to and risk of strength training, offers little additional benefit in strength gains to this population (2, 58). Moreover, it has been reported that one set of moderate-load resistance training is as effective as three sets for increasing bilateral knee extension/flexion strength and muscle size and that this represents a more efficient use of training time (65).

The Training Session

The effectiveness of an exercise program is predicated to a large extent on an appropriate exercise prescription, as well as to sustained compliance. The typical exercise session includes three phases: warm-up, stimulus phase, and cool-down. The remainder of this section provides a brief review of the physiologic basis and rationale for each phase.

Table 1.4   Effects of Lower-Extremity Strength Training on $\dot{V}O_2$max and Endurance During Cycle Ergometer and Treadmill Exercise[*]

	$\dot{V}O_2$max (ml/kg/min)		Endurance (sec)	
	Treadmill	Cycle ergometer	Treadmill	Cycle ergometer
Pretraining	47.8	44.0	291	278
Posttraining	48.8	44.6	325[a]	407[a]

[a]Pretraining vs. posttraining ($p < .01$).
[*]Adapted from Hickson et al. (63).

Warm-Up

The warm-up, including both musculoskeletal and cardiorespiratory activities, prepares the body for the transition from rest to vigorous exercise, increasing blood flow and stretching postural muscles. Moreover, a preliminary warm-up serves to decrease muscle viscosity, susceptibility to injury, and the occurrence of ischemic ST-segment depression and left ventricular dysfunction that may be provoked by sudden strenuous exertion (66, 67). Thus, warm-up has preventive value and enhances performance capacity.

Our experience suggests that the ideal warm-up for any endurance activity is that activity, only at a lower intensity. The cardiorespiratory warm-up should be of sufficient intensity to evoke a heart rate response within 20 beats/min of the minimum heart rate recommended for the stimulus phase. Thus, participants who use slow jogging during this phase might conclude the warm-up period with brisk walking (e.g., 3.5-4.5 mile/hour pace).

Training Stimulus

The stimulus or endurance phase serves to stimulate the oxygen transport system and maximize caloric expenditure. This phase, which may be complemented by resistance training, should be prescribed in terms of specific frequency (how often a person exercises), intensity (how strenuously a person exercises), duration (how long each exercise session is), and mode (the type of exercise that is best). Using an exercise prescription form (see fig. 1.9) is an ideal way of communicating your recommendations to the participant. It is important to remember, however, that interrelationships among these variables may permit a subthreshold level in one factor to be partially or totally compensated for by increases in one or both of the others (19).

Cool-Down

The cool-down consists of a gradual tapering off of intensity after completion of the stimulus phase. It permits appropriate circulatory adjustments and return of the heart rate and blood pressure to near resting values; enhances venous return, thereby reducing the potential for postexercise hypotension; facilitates the dissipation of body heat; and promotes more rapid removal of lactic acid than stationary recovery (68). Exercise should not be halted suddenly but rather should be continued at a modest pace for 5 to 10 minutes, or until the heart rate is substantially reduced and approaches resting values. Cool-down exercises that contract and relax large muscles are suggested because of the massaging effect on the veins, which promotes venous return. Abruptly stopping exercise can cause venous pooling, decreased ventricular filling, and increased myocardial demand due to the postexercise rise in plasma catecholamines (69).

Drug Therapy: Special Considerations for Exercise Testing and Prescription

Cardiac rehabilitation program guidelines should address the need to accommodate changes in medication and dosage adjustments (70, 71). In some instances, repeat exercise testing may be clinically warranted to assess the efficacy of new drug therapy—

MD _____

Name _____ Age _____ Starting date _____

Clinical status: Normal

Arrhythmia   Angina   CABG   CAD   HTN   MI   PTCA   VR

Note: This prescription is valid only if you remain on the same medications (type and dose), and you
are in the same clinical status as on the day your exercise test was conducted.

Contraindications: Angina at rest, fever, illness
Temperature and weather extremes (below 30°F or more than 80°F with high
humidity)

Activities to avoid: Sudden strenuous lifting or carrying
Exertion that leads to holding your breath

Exercise type: Aerobic types of exercise that are continuous, dynamic, and repetitive in nature

Frequency: _____ times/day _____ days/week

Duration: Total duration of exercise session: _____ min

To be divided as follows:

   Warm-up (light flexibility/stretching routine) _____ min

   Aerobic training activity: _____ to _____ min

   Cool-down (slow walking and stretching): _____ min

Intensity:

   Target heart rate _____ to _____ beats/min

   _____ to _____ beats/10 sec

Perceived exertion should not exceed "somewhat hard".

Reevaluation

Your next graded exercise test is due: _____

Call our office to schedule an appointment. Phone: _____

Exercise physiologist: _____

Figure 1.9   Exercise prescription form highlighting individualized recommendations to the
program participant.

for example, with the administration of antiarrhythmic agents. In other situations,
however, exercise testing may not be necessary to revise the prescribed training intensity. Pharmacologic treatment in cardiac exercisers may include

- diuretics,
- beta blockers,
- vasodilators,
- angiotensin-converting enzyme (ACE) inhibitors,
- calcium antagonists (slow channel-blocking agents),
- digitalis,
- antiarrhythmic agents,
- central nervous system-active drugs, and
- alpha-receptor blockers.

The American College of Sports Medicine has extensively reviewed special considerations for exercise prescription (1); here we summarize these considerations briefly.

Diuretics

Under normal circumstances, diuretics do not alter chronotropic reserve or exercise capacity. Thus, prescribed heart rates and work rates for exercise training generally remain unchanged (1). Such therapy, however, can cause hypokalemia, muscle fatigue, ventricular arrhythmias, and, occasionally, spurious ST-segment depression (72).

Beta Blockers

Beta blocker therapy reduces submaximal and maximal heart rate, blood pressure, cardiac output, muscle blood flow, and, frequently, exercise capacity. The decrease in physical work capacity and/or ability to sustain submaximal exercise may be even greater with nonselective than with cardioselective agents (73, 74), perhaps because the nonselective agents impair utilization of carbohydrates (75). On the other hand, patients with angina who are taking beta blockers may achieve a higher functional capacity with less ST-segment depression and reduced symptoms at submaximal and maximal exercise.

Although one earlier review suggested that beta blockade may attenuate desired training benefits (76), several other studies have shown that patients may derive considerable physiologic benefit from a physical conditioning program in the presence of both cardioselective and nonselective beta-blocking drugs, despite therapeutic doses and a reduced training heart rate (77-79). Because beta blockers do not alter the remarkably consistent relationship between oxygen consumption ($\dot{V}O_2$) and heart rate, expressed as percentages of their respective maximal values, it appears that the generally accepted metabolic load for training (60-80% $\dot{V}O_2$max), associated with favorable adaptation and improvement, may be achieved by patients on beta blockade at the conventional relative heart rate recommendation for training (70-85% HRmax) (80).

If beta blocker therapy is decreased or discontinued, repeat exercise testing is often recommended in cardiac exercisers to assess signs or symptoms of myocardial ischemia and/or arrhythmias that may have been previously camouflaged. In contrast, if the beta blocker dosage is increased, repeat exercise testing may not be necessary to adjust the training intensity. Because functional capacity generally remains unchanged, the exercise leader may simply assess the reduced heart rate response to the patient's usual training work rates and establish this as the "new" target heart rate, using perceived exertion as an adjunct intensity guide. The concept of perceived exertion appears to be valid for patients whose heart rates are attenuated by beta blockade, since similar ratings are obtained at a given percentage of maximum heart rate reserve regardless of the beta blocker dosage or peak heart rate (38).

For patients on "long-acting" beta blockers, prescription of the target heart rate should be based on the results of an exercise test that is conducted at approximately the same time of day the subject will be exercising, as the significant reduction in heart rate response may dissipate over time. To test this hypothesis, we subjected 18 cardiac patients on low-dose (50 mg) atenolol QD to morning and late-afternoon exercise testing (Bruce protocol) (81). Although mean exercise time for morning versus afternoon testing was not significantly different (11.2 vs. 11.5 min), peak exercise heart rates during afternoon testing were uniformly higher (range, 5 to 35 beats/min; $\bar{x} = 20$ beats/min; $p < .001$), as were the double products, 272 versus 208 mmHg × beats/min × 10^{-2}. There were no ischemic ECGs during morning exercise testing. In contrast, 5 of 18 patients (28%) demonstrated ST-segment depression equal to or greater than 1 mm during afternoon testing. Thus, prescribed exercise heart rates for patients on once-daily beta blockers may be inaccurate unless the exercise testing and training time are similar.

Vasodilators

Because vasodilators do not generally modify the heart rate response to submaximal and maximal work rates, exercise intensity can be based on conventional prescriptive methods, obviating the need for repeat exercise testing (1). These agents, however, can increase exercise capacity in patients with angina pectoris or heart failure.

Angiotensin-Converting Enzyme Inhibitors

Because ACE inhibitors decrease blood pressure at rest and during exercise without influencing other adaptational mechanisms such as heart rate and cardiac output (82), training intensity may be prescribed in the usual manner (1). ACE inhibitors may increase exercise capacity in patients with chronic heart failure.

Calcium Antagonists

In contrast to beta blockers, calcium antagonists do not generally impair cardiac output, muscle blood flow, functional capacity, or exercise trainability (83-86). However, certain calcium channel blockers can decrease the heart rate and blood pressure responses at a given external work rate, delay the time to ischemia, and improve exercise capacity. Verapamil, for example, tends to have a negative chronotropic effect (71). Consequently one should base the prescribed heart rate for training on the medicated patient's individual response to an exercise test (1).

Digitalis

Aside from its use in the treatment of atrial fibrillation, digitalis appears to have little effect on the hemodynamic and metabolic responses to exercise. ST-segment depression can be induced or accentuated during exercise in persons with or without heart disease who are taking digitalis (87). In patients taking digitalis, profound ST-segment depression may indicate myocardial ischemia, particularly when it is accompanied by a prolonged QT interval (1). Nevertheless, exercise induced ST-segment depression should be interpreted with caution in the presence of digitalis therapy, and additional studies (e.g., with concomitant myocardial perfusion imaging) may be used to differentiate true- and false-positive responses.

Because exercise-induced ST-segment depression may persist after digoxin is discontinued, it is best to wait at least 10-14 days before "diagnostic" exercise testing, provided there are no strong clinical contraindications to withholding the drug (88).

Antiarrhythmic Agents

Although quinidine can diminish the magnitude of ST-segment depression, it does not change the heart rate or aerobic capacity in normal subjects or in patients with CAD. In contrast, a decrease of 20 beats/min in maximum exercise heart rate has been reported in patients taking amiodarone.

Central Nervous System-Active Drugs

Agents that act on the central nervous system, including clonidine, guanfacine, and guanabenz, can have attenuating effects on the heart rate and blood pressure during exercise. Because the hemodynamic responses to physical activity may vary considerably, one should formulate exercise guidelines conservatively and should carefully monitor the potential for adverse reactions, including hypotension, dizziness, and syncope.

Alpha-Receptor Blockers

Although alpha-receptor blockers effectively lower systolic and diastolic blood pressure, they appear to have negligible effects on heart rate, cardiac output, and metabolic responses to exercise. For patients on these agents, therefore, one can prescribe training in the usual manner, using heart rate as an indicator of exercise intensity.

Safety of Exercise-Based Cardiac Rehabilitation

According to 1980-1984 survey data, the incidence of cardiovascular complications was one cardiac arrest per 111,996 patient-hours, one acute myocardial infarction per 292,990 patient-hours, and one fatality in 783,972 patient-hours of exercise-based cardiac rehabilitation (89). However, this low mortality rate applies only to medically supervised programs equipped with a defibrillator and appropriate emergency drugs. Up to 90% of all patients with cardiac arrest occurring under such conditions were successfully resuscitated.

High-Intensity Training as a Trigger for Acute Cardiac Events

Untoward events during exercise training are more likely to occur among cardiac patients than among presumably healthy adults. For patients with CAD, the relative risk of developing cardiac arrest during vigorous exercise is estimated to be 6 to 164 times greater than at rest or during light activity (90). Exertion-related cardiac arrest is typically due to an arrhythmic event such as ventricular fibrillation rather than to acute myocardial infarction.

Pathophysiologic evidence suggests that vigorous physical exertion, by increasing myocardial oxygen consumption and simultaneously shortening diastole and coronary perfusion time, may evoke a transient oxygen deficiency at the subendocardial level, which can be exacerbated by a decreased venous return secondary to abrupt cessation of activity (see fig. 1.10). Ischemia can alter depolarization, repolarization, and conduction velocity, triggering serious ventricular arrhythmias, which in extreme

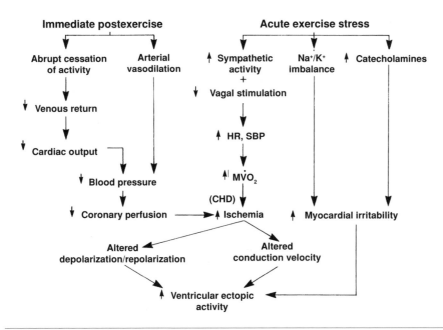

Figure 1.10   Physiologic alterations accompanying acute exercise and recovery, and their possible sequelae. CHD, coronary heart disease; HR, heart rate; MV̇O$_2$, myocardial oxygen uptake; Na$^+$/K$^+$, sodium/potassium ion; SBP, systolic blood pressure.

cases may be the harbingers of ventricular tachycardia or fibrillation. In addition, symptomatic or silent myocardial ischemia (5), sodium-potassium imbalance, increased catecholamine excretion, and circulating free fatty acids all may be arrhythmogenic.

Two recent studies, one in the United States (91) and the other in Germany (92), reported that the "relative risk" of acute myocardial infarction during or soon after strenuous physical exertion ($\geq$ 6 METs) was two to six times greater than the risk during periods of lighter activity or no exertion. The reason may be that abrupt increases in heart rate and blood pressure give rise to hemodynamic stresses that disrupt vulnerable atherosclerotic plaque and lead to thrombotic occlusion of a coronary vessel. However, the relative risk varied greatly depending on the patient's usual frequency of physical activity. In the German study, patients who exercised less than four times per week and those who exercised four times or more per week had relative risks of 6.9 and 1.3, respectively. The U.S. study revealed that among persons who usually exercised less than one time per week, one to two times per week, three to four times per week, and five or more times per week, the respective relative risks were 107, 19.4, 8.6, and 2.4. Thus, both studies concluded that regular exercise provides protection against the triggering of acute myocardial infarction by strenuous exertion.

Factors Affecting Safety

The safety of regimens of high-intensity exercise training has been challenged in retrospective reports of patients with CAD who developed cardiovascular complications during or shortly after medically supervised rehabilitation exercise (93, 94). Patients with previous myocardial infarction who have impaired left ventricular function, significant exercise-induced ST-segment depression, angina pectoris, threatening ventricular arrhythmias, or an above-average functional capacity appear to be at increased risk of untoward events. Individuals who have had a cardiac arrest are also more likely to disregard appropriate warm-up and cool-down procedures or exhibit poor compliance to the prescribed training heart rate range (i.e., exercise-intensity violators). These and other recent data (95) suggest that unconventionally vigorous exercise is associated with an increased risk of cardiovascular complications in selected patients with CAD.

Effects of Exercise-Based Cardiac Rehabilitation

Exercise training appears to play an important role in the medical management and rehabilitation of patients with CAD. The salutary effects of chronic exercise training are well documented.

Benefits of Exercise Training

Common rationale for exercise training of patients with CAD include increases in aerobic capacity and relief of symptoms of myocardial ischemia. Favorable risk factor modification, improved psychosocial well-being, and increased survival are also expected outcomes.

Aerobic Capacity

The increase in $\dot{V}O_2$max in patients with CAD varies inversely with the pretraining $\dot{V}O_2$max and ranges from 11% to 56% (mean = 20%) after 3 months of endurance exercise training (96). Improved aerobic capacity, which is commonly attributed to increases in the maximal arteriovenous oxygen difference, and in some cases stroke volume as well, is particularly beneficial, since most patients with clinically manifest heart disease have a subnormal $\dot{V}O_2$max (50-70% age, gender predicted). Because a given submaximal task or work rate has a relatively constant aerobic requirement, cardiac patients find that after a physical conditioning program, they are working at a lower percentage of their aerobic capacity, with greater reserve (see fig. 1.11).

Relief of Symptoms

The potential value of exercise therapy in relieving anginal symptoms was recognized almost as early as the clinical description of heart disease itself. In 1772, Herberden noted that one of his symptomatic patients was "nearly cured" after 6 months of sawing wood on a regular basis. Today it is generally recognized that some of the greatest increases in exercise tolerance following physical training occur in patients with angina on exertion (2). Reductions in myocardial oxygen demand via decreases in two of its major determinants, heart rate alone or the heart rate-systolic blood pressure product, are largely responsible (96). Decreased myocardial oxygen demands presumably allow the cardiac patient to exercise at higher work intensities

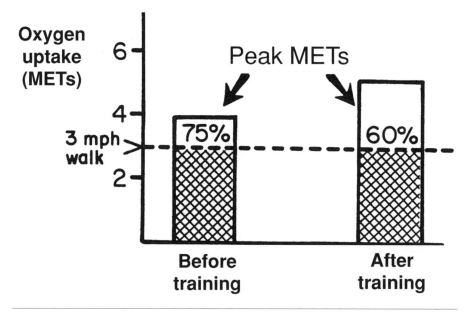

Figure 1.11   Effect of exercise training on peak oxygen uptake (METs) and relative oxygen cost (activity METs/peak METs) of walking at 3 mph on a level grade. Following a physical conditioning program, peak oxygen uptake increased from 4 to 5 METs, decreasing the relative oxygen cost of a 3 mph walk from 75% to 60%.

before reaching the critical rate-pressure product at which symptoms occur (anginal threshold). Improvements in coronary blood flow may be related, at least in part, to the decreased heart rate at rest and during submaximal exercise. Because coronary blood flow predominates in diastole, coronary perfusion time is increased. Thus, a conditioning bradycardia appears to play a critical role in prevention of ischemia and relief of symptoms in patients with CAD.

Coronary Risk Factors

Aerobic exercise training, especially when incorporated as part of a *multifactorial* intervention, can result in modest decreases in body weight, fat stores, and blood pressure (particularly in hypertensives). A meta-analysis of statistically aggregated data from 15 longitudinal studies of the effect of moderate exercise training in 490 male post-myocardial infarction patients has demonstrated significant alterations in lipids and lipoproteins (97). Triglyceride levels decreased from 169 mg/dl to 149 mg/dl; total cholesterol levels decreased from 232 mg/dl to 221 mg/dl; low-density lipoprotein cholesterol levels decreased from 145 mg/dl to 140 mg/dl; and the "antiatherogenic" high-density lipoprotein cholesterol subfraction increased from 41 mg/dl to 45 mg/dl with training.

Psychosocial Well-Being

Exercise training may improve well-being and self-efficacy in some cardiac patients, especially in the performance of physical tasks. Some investigators have reported an improved quality of life and reduced depression in clinically depressed post-myocardial infarction patients following exercise-based cardiac rehabilitation programs (2). However, most randomized, controlled trials of exercise training suggest less impressive effects in modulating the psychosocial dysfunction complicating acute coronary events (19). Thus, it appears that group therapy or stress management may be more effective interventions than exercise training for improving psychosocial well-being.

Morbidity and Mortality

Eight of the major randomized trials of rehabilitation with exercise after myocardial infarction (see table 1.5) involved a total of 3,103 patients who were followed for 1 to 9 years (98-105). Effectiveness of these interventions, as expressed by the formula [(control mortality–intervention mortality/control mortality) $\times$ 100], showed a beneficial trend toward increased survival (7 of 8 trials), but the results in only one study (102) attained statistical significance. Because these studies were limited by sample size, recent attempts have been made to pool data from similar randomized clinical trials.

Three meta-analyses (106-108) have now shown that exercise-based cardiac rehabilitation provides a 20-25% reduction in total and cardiovascular-related mortality, with no difference in the rate of nonfatal recurrent events. The exercise dosage in these studies generally ranged from 50% to 75% $\dot{V}O_2$max for 20 to 60 minutes, two to four times per week, suggesting that the reduction in fatal cardiac events after cardiac rehabilitation may be achieved with mild-to-moderate exercise intensities. These results, however, cannot necessarily be extrapolated to patients following coronary artery bypass graft surgery and/or percutaneous transluminal coronary angioplasty (109). In addition, contemporary thrombolytic and revascularization procedures, which markedly decrease early postinfarction mortality, would likely diminish the impact of adjunctive exercise-based cardiac rehabilitation programs on survival (2).

Table 1.5   Cardiac Rehabilitation Trial Results

Trials	Reference number	Mortality (%) Control	Mortality (%) Intervention	Effectiveness (%)
Sanne	(98)	23	18	22
Hakkila	(99)	12	10	15
Kentala	(100)	22	17	22
Palatsi	(101)	14	10	29
Kallio	(102)	30	22	27
Shaw	(103)	7	5	37
Shephard	(104)	7	10	−30
Roman	(105)	6	4*	38

*Mortality expressed in percentage per year of patients followed up.

Relation Between Fitness and All-Cause Mortality

Blair et al. (110) showed that a low level of aerobic fitness, expressed as metabolic equivalents (METs; 1 MET = 3.5 ml O_2/kg/min), is an independent risk factor for all-cause mortality. In general, the higher the initial level of fitness, the lower was the subsequent death rate from cancer and heart disease (see fig. 1.12), even after statistical adjustments were made for age, risk factors, and family history of heart disease. Interestingly, there appeared to be no additional benefit (i.e., lower mortality) associated with fitness levels higher than 9 to 10 METs. The greatest reduction in risk occurred as one progressed from the lowest level of fitness ($\leq$ 6 METs) to the next lowest level (7 METs), suggesting that even a modest improvement in fitness among the most unfit confers a substantial health benefit. The investigators emphasized that the fitness levels associated with a plateau in death rates, 9 to 10 METs, can be attained by most men and women who walk briskly on a regular basis. These findings and other recent reports have confirmed an inverse association between physical fitness and cardiovascular mortality.

Recently, Blair and coworkers (111) reported on the relationship between *changes* in aerobic fitness and the risk of death in men. The highest death rate (122.0/10,000 man-years) occurred in men who were unfit at both examinations; the lowest death rate (39.6/10,000 man-years) was in men who were physically fit at both examinations. Men who improved from the unfit to the fit category between the first and

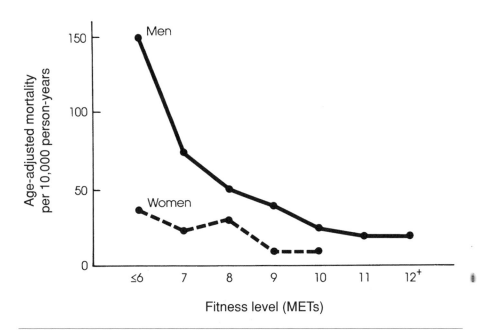

Figure 1.12   Age-adjusted, all-cause mortality rates per 10,000 person-years of follow-up by aerobic fitness (METs) achieved during maximal treadmill exercise testing. Adapted from Blair et al. (110).

second examinations had an intermediate death rate (67.7/10,000 man-years), even after adjustments were made for age, health status, and other risk factors. For each minute increase in treadmill time between examinations, there was a 7.9% decrease ($p = .001$) in risk of mortality. These important new findings support a *cause-and-effect relationship* between improved aerobic fitness and reduced mortality, rather than merely an association between these variables.

Limitations of Exercise Training

Although the benefits that exercise training offers in secondary prevention are undeniable, there are limitations. Contrary to the speculation of a few overzealous enthusiasts, regular exercise training, regardless of the dosage, does not necessarily prevent progression of CAD or, for that matter, restenosis or reinfarction. Conventional exercise training also does little to increase left ventricular ejection fraction and myocardial perfusion. Numerous training studies have now demonstrated increased exercise tolerance in patients with impaired left ventricular function (ejection fraction < 45%), despite the lack of improvement in resting hemodynamics or ejection fraction. Attempts to use myocardial perfusion imaging (e.g., thallium-201 exercise testing) before and after physical training have produced conflicting and often unremarkable findings, whereas angiographic studies in group trials have without exception yielded disappointing results. Thus, direct evidence that exercise increases coronary collateralization or vessel diameter, or that it reverses coronary narrowing, is lacking (2, 19, 109).

The Compliance Problem

Although many patients can be encouraged to initiate an exercise-training program, favorable physiologic and clinical outcomes result only from continued participation. Unfortunately, negative variables often outweigh the positive variables contributing to sustained participant interest and enthusiasm (see fig. 1.13). Such imbalance often leads to a decline in adherence, diminishing program effectiveness. Adult fitness and exercise-based cardiac rehabilitation programs have reported average dropout rates of 46% and 44%, respectively, highlighting the compliance problem among those who voluntarily enter physical conditioning programs (see fig. 1.14) (112). Thus, it appears that exercise is not unlike other health-related behaviors (e.g., medication compliance, smoking cessation, weight reduction) in that *typically half or less of those who initiate the behavior will continue,* irrespective of initial health status or type of program.

Research and empiric experience suggest that certain program modifications and motivational strategies may enhance patient enrollment, interest, and compliance (112, 113). These strategies include the following:

- **Recruiting physician support of the cardiac exercise program.** According to one recent study (114), the single most important factor determining a patient's participation in an exercise-based cardiac rehabilitation program was receiving a strong recommendation from his/her primary care physician.

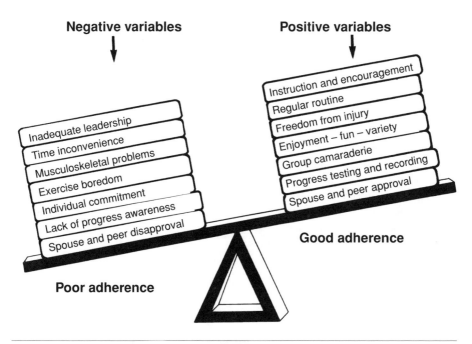

Figure 1.13   Variables affecting adherence to an exercise-training program.

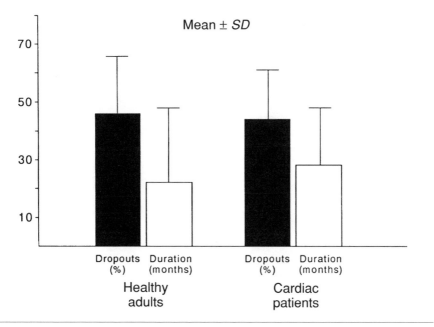

Figure 1.14   Relationship between the dropout rate (%) and the duration of exercise training (months) in healthy adults and cardiac patients.

- **Establishing short-term goals.** Patients should be oriented to short-term objectives that are specific, clearly defined, and realistically attainable, based on their particular stage of readiness for change (115). In other words, individuals progress in a sequence of stages along a continuum of behavioral change from not intending to make changes (precontemplation), to considering a change (contemplation), to making small changes (preparation), to actively engaging in the new behavior (action), to sustaining the change over time (maintenance). There is also the possibility of recidivism, that is, relapse back to an earlier stage. Interventions that are specifically targeted to the patient's stage of readiness for change, as established during the postevaluation consult, are more likely to further the patient's momentum in the direction of permanent lifestyle change.
- **Minimizing injury/complications with a mild-to-moderate exercise prescription.** Often, novice exercisers become discouraged due to muscular soreness or orthopedic injury from increasing the activity dosage too abruptly. Excessive exercise frequency ($\geq$5 days/week), duration ($\geq$45 min/session), and/or intensity (>90% $\dot{V}O_2max$) offer the patient little additional gain in aerobic fitness, yet the incidence of injury

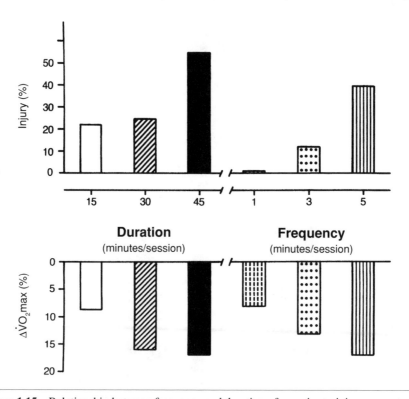

Figure 1.15   Relationship between frequency and duration of exercise training, percentage improvement in aerobic capacity ($\Delta\dot{V}O_2max$), and the incidence of orthopedic injury. Above an exercise duration of 30 minutes/session, or a frequency of 3 sessions/week, additional improvement in $\dot{V}O_2max$ is small, yet the incidence of injury increases disproportionately. Adapted from Pollock et al. (41).

increases markedly (see fig. 1.15) (41). A recommended program for beginners is to walk 20 to 30 minutes every other day at a perceived exertion (6-20 scale) of 11 to 13, corresponding to "fairly light" to "somewhat hard." Patients should also be counseled to discontinue exercise and seek medical advice if they experience anginal discomfort or dizziness.

- **Encouraging group participation.** Commitments made as part of a group tend to be stronger than those made independently. The social support and camaraderie of the group often provide the incentive to continue during periods of sagging interest or enthusiasm.
- **Emphasizing fun and variety in the exercise program.** Regimented calisthenics, when relied on too heavily in an exercise program, become monotonous and boring, leading to poor exercise adherence. The most successful physical conditioning programs are those that are pleasurable and that offer the greatest diversification.
- **Providing positive reinforcement through periodic fitness testing.** Exercise testing, body fatness assessment, and serum lipid profiling should be performed at program entry and at regular intervals thereafter in order to assess an individual's response to the exercise stimulus. Improvements in these evaluations can serve as powerful motivators that produce renewed interest and dedication.
- **Recruiting spouse support of the exercise program.** A participant's spouse, as well as family and friends, can also influence exercise compliance. The importance of this influence became apparent in one study that showed a direct relationship between the husband's adherence to the exercise program and the wife's attitude toward it (see fig. 1.16) (116). Of those men whose spouse had a positive attitude toward the program, 80% demonstrated a good to excellent adherence pattern. However, when the spouses' attitudes were neutral or negative, only 40% showed good to excellent adherence patterns.
- **Including an optional recreational game in the exercise program format.** A recreational game is recommended to complement the standard cardiac exercise program. However, game rules should be modified to minimize skill and competition and maximize participant success.
- **Increasing access to the training facility.** Availability of morning and afternoon exercise sessions at least every other day (ideally 5-6 days/week) should serve to further increase the compatibility of an exercise commitment with the varied schedules of participants.
- **Using progress charts to record exercise achievements.** A progress chart or computer-based documentation that allows participants to record daily exercise achievements provides immediate positive feedback and reinforcement of activity-related behaviors.
- **Recognizing individual accomplishments.** Peer recognition is a powerful motivator. To this end, an annual awards ceremony or banquet is recommended. Recognition of participant accomplishments can take the form of inexpensive trophies, plaques, ribbons, or certificates.
- **Providing qualified, enthusiastic exercise leaders.** Although numerous variables affect exercise adherence, perhaps the single most important is the exercise leader.

Positive

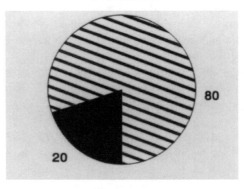

Neutral or negative

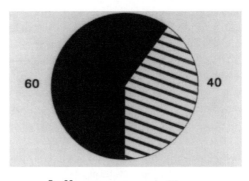

Adherence patterns

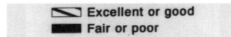

Figure 1.16   Relation of wives' attitudes to husbands' adherence to an exercise training program. Adapted from Heinzelman and Bagley (116).

Exercise leaders should be well trained, highly motivated, compassionate, tactful, innovative, and enthusiastic. Workshop and certification offerings by the American College of Sports Medicine and other professional organizations serve to promote "quality control" and knowledge and proficiency standards for program personnel.

Conclusions

The exercise prescription consists of intensity, duration, frequency, and mode of training, and is based on the results of a comprehensive patient evaluation. For optimal outcomes, the exercise prescription should be individualized and periodically adjusted so that the overload principle is continually evoked. Training adaptation usually begins in about 4 to 6 weeks, although the rate of improvement varies widely among individuals. One must consider the principle of training specificity as well as individual needs, interests, motivation, clinical status, and concomitant drug therapy in designing the prescription and training program. Appropriately prescribed exercise-training programs for cardiac patients are associated with extremely low complication rates and numerous health benefits. Although exercise guidelines should be developed as scientifically as possible, the exercise prescription should be adapted to the patient, rather than the patient to the prescription.

References

1. American College of Sports Medicine. *Guidelines for exercise testing and prescription*, 5th ed. Baltimore: Williams & Wilkins; 1995.
2. Wenger, N.K., Froelicher, E.S., Smith, L.K., et al. *Cardiac rehabilitation as secondary prevention. Clinical practice guideline. Quick reference guide for clinicians,* No. 17. Rockville, MD: U.S. Department of Health and Human Services, Public Health Service, Agency for Health Care Policy and Research and National Heart, Lung, and Blood Institute. AHCPR Pub. No. 96-0673; October 1995.
3. Myers, J., and Froelicher, V.F. Predicting outcome in cardiac rehabilitation. *Journal of the American College of Cardiology,* **15**, 983-985; 1990.
4. Hess, O.M., Schneider, J., Nonogi, H., et al. Myocardial structure in patients with exercise-induced ischemia. *Circulation,* **77**, 967-977; 1988.
5. Hoberg, E., Schuler, G., Kunze, B., et al. Silent myocardial ischemia as a potential link between lack of premonitoring symptoms and increased risk of cardiac arrest during physical stress. *American Journal of Cardiology,* **65**, 583-589; 1990.
6. Jugdutt, B.I., Michorowski, B.L., and Kappagoda, C.T. Exercise training after anterior Q wave myocardial infarction: importance of regional left ventricular function and topography. *Journal of the American College of Cardiology,* **12**, 362-372; 1988.
7. Mark, D.B., Hlatky, M.A., Califf, R.M., et al. Painless exercise ST deviation on the treadmill: long-term prognosis. *Journal of the American College of Cardiology,* **14**, 885-892; 1989.
8. Schuler, G., Shlierf, G., Wirth, A., et al. Low fat diet and regular, supervised physical exercise in patients with symptomatic coronary artery disease: reduction of stress-induced myocardial ischemia. *Circulation,* **77**, 172-181; 1988.
9. Sullivan, M.J., Higginbotham, M.B., and Cobb, F.R. Exercise training in patients with severe left ventricular dysfunction: hemodynamic and metabolic effects. *Circulation,* **78**, 506-515; 1988.
10. Giannuzzi, P., Temporelli, P.L., Tavazzi, L., et al. EAMI-exercise training in anterior myocardial infarction: an ongoing multicenter randomized study; preliminary results on left ventricular function and remodeling. *Chest,* **101**(5 Suppl.):315S-321S; 1992.

11. Giannuzzi, P., Tavazzi, L., Temporelli, P.L., et al. Long-term physical training and left ventricular remodeling after anterior myocardial infarction: results of the Exercise in Anterior Myocardial Infarction (EAMI) trial. *Journal of the American College of Cardiology,* **22**, 1821-1829; 1993.

12. Fardy, P.S., Yanowitz, F.G., and Wilson, P.K. *Cardiac rehabilitation, adult fitness, and exercise testing,* 3rd ed. Philadelphia: Lea & Febiger; 1995.

13. Fardy, P.S., Webb, D., and Hellerstein, H.K. Benefits of arm exercise in cardiac rehabilitation. *Physician and Sportsmedicine,* **5**, 30-41; 1977.

14. Buskirk, E., and Taylor, H.L. Maximal oxygen intake and its relation to body composition, with special reference to chronic physical activity and obesity. *Journal of Applied Physiology,* **2**, 72-78; 1957.

15. Franklin, B.A. Pitfalls in estimating aerobic capacity from exercise time or workload. *Applied Cardiology,* **14**, 25-26; 1986.

16. Sullivan, M., and McKirnan, M.D. Errors in predicting functional capacity for postmyocardial infarction patients using a modified Bruce protocol. *American Heart Journal,* **107**, 486-492; 1984.

17. Hughson, R.L., and Smyth, G.A. Slower adaptation of $\dot{V}O_2$ to steady-state of submaximal exercise with beta-adrenergic blockade. *European Journal of Applied Physiology,* **52**, 107-110; 1983.

18. Franklin, B.A. Easy does it for health. *Fitness Management,* **9**, 41-43; 1993.

19. Franklin, B.A., Gordon, S., and Timmis, G.C. Amount of exercise necessary for the patient with coronary artery disease. *American Journal of Cardiology,* **69**, 1426-1432; 1992.

20. Wilmore, J.H. Exercise prescription: role of the physiatrist and allied health professional. *Archives of Physical Medicine and Rehabilitation,* **57**, 15-19; 1976.

21. Wilmore, J.H., and Haskell, W. Use of the heart rate-energy expenditure relationship in the individual prescription of exercise. *American Journal of Clinical Nutrition,* **24**, 1186-1192; 1971.

22. Hellerstein, H.K., Hirsch, E.Z., Ader, R., et al. Principles of exercise prescription for normals and cardiac subjects. In: Naughton, J.P., Hellerstein, H.K., and Mohler, I.C. eds. *Exercise testing and exercise training in coronary heart disease.* New York: Academic Press; 1973:pp. 129-167.

23. Taylor, H.L., Haskell, W., Fox, S.M. III, et al. Exercise tests: a summary of procedures and concepts of stress testing for cardiovascular diagnosis and function evaluation. In: Blackburn, H., ed. *Measurement in exercise electrocardiography* (the Ernst Simonson Conference). Springfield, IL: Charles C Thomas; 1969:pp. 259-305.

24. Hossack, K.F., Bruce, R.A., and Clark, L.J. Influence of propranolol on exercise prescription of training heart rates. *Cardiology,* **65**, 47-58; 1980.

25. Franklin, B., Hodgson, H., and Buskirk, E.R. Relationship between percent maximal O_2 uptake and percent maximal heart rate in women. *Research Quarterly for Exercise and Sport,* **51**, 616-624; 1980.

26. Karvonen, M., Kentala, K., and Mustala, O. The effects of training on heart rate: a longitudinal study. *Annales Medicinae Experimentalis et Biologiae Fenniae,* **35**, 307-315; 1957.

27. Davis, J.A., and Convertino, J.A. A comparison of heart rate methods for predicting endurance training intensity. *Medicine and Science in Sports,* **7**, 295-298; 1975.
28. Dressendorfer, R.H., and Smith, J.L. Predictive accuracy of the maximum heart rate reserve method for estimating aerobic training intensity in early cardiac rehabilitation. *Journal of Cardiac Rehabilitation,* **4**, 484-489; 1984.
29. Fox, S.M., Naughton, J.P., and Haskell, W.L. Physical activity and the prevention of coronary heart disease. *Annals of Clinical Research,* **3**, 404-432; 1971.
30. Dressendorfer, R.H., Franklin, B.A., Gordon, S., and Timmis, G.C. Resting oxygen uptake in coronary artery disease: influence of chronic beta blockade. *Chest,* **104**, 1269-1272; 1993.
31. Pandolf, K.B., Cafarelli, E., Noble, B.J., et al. Hyperthermia: effect on exercise prescription. *Archives of Physical Medicine and Rehabilitation,* **56**, 524-526; 1975.
32. Franklin, B.A., and Hellerstein, H.K. Realistic stress testing for activity prescription. *Journal of Cardiovascular Medicine,* **7**, 570-576; 1982.
33. Kitamura, K., Jorgensen, C.R., Gobel, F.L., et al. Hemodynamic correlates of myocardial oxygen consumption during upright exercise. *Journal of Applied Physiology,* **32**, 516-522; 1972.
34. Nelson, R.R., Gobel, F.L., Jorgensen, C.R., et al. Hemodynamic predictors of myocardial oxygen consumption during static and dynamic exercise. *Circulation,* **50**, 1179-1189; 1974.
35. Squires, R.S. Rehabilitation after cardiac transplantation: 1980-1990. *Journal of Cardiopulmonary Rehabilitation,* **11**, 84-92; 1991.
36. Squires, R.W. Cardiac rehabilitation issues for heart transplantation patients. *Journal of Cardiopulmonary Rehabilitation,* **10**, 159-168; 1990.
37. Borg, G. Psychophysical bases of perceived exertion. *Medicine and Science in Sports and Exercise,* **14**, 377-381; 1982.
38. Pollock, M.L., Lowenthal, D.T., Foster, C., et al. Acute and chronic responses to exercise in patients treated with beta blockers. *Journal of Cardiopulmonary Rehabilitation,* **11**, 132-144; 1991.
39. Williams, M.A., and Fardy, P.S. Limitations in prescribing exercise. *Journal of Cardiovascular and Pulmonary Technique,* **8**, 36-38; 1980.
40. Dressendorfer, R.H., Franklin, B.A., Cameron, J.L., et al. Exercise training frequency in early post-infarction cardiac rehabilitation: influence on aerobic conditioning. *Journal of Cardiopulmonary Rehabilitation,* **15**, 269-276; 1995.
41. Pollock, M.L., Gettman, L.R., Milesis, C.A., et al. Effects of frequency and duration of training on attrition and incidence of injury. *Medicine and Science in Sports,* **9**, 31-36; 1977.
42. Fardy, P.S., and Ilmarinen, J. Evaluating the effects and feasibility of an at work stairclimbing intervention program for men. *Medicine and Science in Sports,* **7**, 91-93; 1975.
43. Pollock, M.L., and Wilmore, J.H. *Exercise in health and disease,* 2nd ed. Philadelphia: W.B. Saunders Company; 1990.
44. DeBusk, R.F., Stenestrand, U., Sheehan, M., et al. Training effects of long versus short bouts of exercise in healthy subjects. *American Journal of Cardiology,* **65**, 1010-1013; 1990.

45. Shaw, L.W. Effects of a prescribed supervised exercise program on mortality and cardiovascular morbidity in patients after a myocardial infarction. *American Journal of Cardiology,* **48**, 39-46; 1981.
46. Fardy, P.S. Isometric exercise and the cardiovascular system. *Physician and Sportsmedicine,* **9**, 43-56; 1981.
47. Clausen, J.P., Trap-Jensen, J., and Lassen, N.A. The effects of training on the heart rate during arm and leg exercise. *Scandinavian Journal of Clinical and Laboratory Investigation,* **26**, 295-301; 1970.
48. Klausen, K., Rasmussen, B., Clausen, J.P., et al. Blood lactate from exercising extremities before and after arm or leg training. *American Journal of Physiology,* **227**, 67-72; 1974.
49. Rasmussen, B., Klausen, K., Clausen, J.P., et al. Pulmonary ventilation, blood gases and blood pH after training of the arms or the legs. *Journal of Applied Physiology,* **38**, 250-256; 1975.
50. Henriksson, J., and Reitman, J.S. Time course of changes in human skeletal muscle succinate dehydrogenase and cytochrome oxidase activities and maximal oxygen uptake with physical activity and inactivity. *Acta Physiologica Scandinavia,* **99**, 91-97; 1977.
51. Fardy, P.S., Doll, N.E., Reitz, N.L., et al. Prevalence of dysrhythmias during upper, lower and combined upper and lower extremity exercise in cardiac patients [abstract]. *Medicine and Science in Sports,* **13**, 137; 1981.
52. Franklin, B.A., Vander, L., Wrisley, D., et al. Trainability of arms versus legs in men with previous myocardial infarction. *Chest,* **105**, 262-264; 1994.
53. Franklin, B.A. Exercise testing, training and arm ergometry. *Sports Medicine,* **2**, 100-119; 1985.
54. Franklin, B.A., Vander, L., Wrisley, D., et al. Aerobic requirements of arm ergometry: implications for exercise testing and training. *Physician and Sportsmedicine,* **11**, 81-90; 1983.
55. Wetherbee, S., Franklin, B.A., Hollingsworth, V., et al. Relationship between arm and leg training work loads in men with heart disease: implications for exercise prescription. *Chest,* **99**, 1271-1273; 1991.
56. Makalous, S.L., Araujo, J., and Thomas, T.R. Energy expenditure during walking with hand weights. *Physician and Sportsmedicine,* **16**, 139-148; 1988.
57. DeBusk, R.F., Pitts, W., Haskell, W., et al. Comparison of cardiovascular responses to static-dynamic and dynamic effort alone in patients with ischemic heart disease. *Circulation,* **59**, 977-984; 1979.
58. Franklin, B.A., Bonzheim, K., Gordon, S., et al. Resistance training in cardiac rehabilitation. *Journal of Cardiopulmonary Rehabilitation,* **11**, 99-107; 1991.
59. Lind, A.R., and McNichol, G.W. Muscular factors which determine the cardiovascular responses to sustained and rhythmic exercise. *Canadian Medical Association Journal,* **96**, 706-715; 1967.
60. Mitchell, J.H., Payne, F.C., Saltin, B., et al. The role of muscle mass in the cardiovascular response to static contractions. *Journal of Physiology,* **309**, 45-54; 1980.
61. Pollock, M.L., Wilmore, J.H., and Fox, S.M. *Health and fitness through physical activity.* New York: Wiley; 1978:p. 45.

62. Lewis, S., Nygaard, E., Sanchez, J., et al. Static contraction of the quadriceps muscle in man: cardiovascular control and responses to one-legged strength training. *Acta Physiologica Scandinavia,* **122**, 341-353; 1984.

63. Hickson, R.C., Rosenkoetter, M.A., and Brown, M.M. Strength training effects on aerobic power and short-term endurance. *Medicine and Science in Sports and Exercise,* **12**, 336-339; 1980.

64. Goldberg, L., Elliot, D.L., Schutz, R.W., et al. Changes in lipid and lipoprotein levels after weight training. *Journal of the American Medical Association,* **252**, 504-506; 1984.

65. Starkey, D.B., Pollock, M.L., Ishida, Y., et al. Effect of resistance training volume on strength and muscle thickness. *Medicine and Science in Sports and Exercise,* **28**, 1311-1320,1996.

66. Barnard, R.J., Gardner, G.W., Diaco, N.V., et al. Cardiovascular responses to sudden strenuous exercise: heart rate, blood pressure, and ECG. *Journal of Applied Physiology,* **34**, 833-837; 1973.

67. Foster, C., Anholm, J.D., Hellman, C.K., et al. Left ventricular function during sudden strenuous exercise. *Circulation,* **63**, 592-596; 1981.

68. Belcastro, A.N., and Bonen, A. Lactic acid removal rates during controlled and uncontrolled recovery exercise. *Journal of Applied Physiology,* **39**, 932-936; 1975.

69. Dimsdale, J.E., Hartley, H., Guiney, T., et al. Postexercise peril: plasma catecholamines and exercise. *Journal of the American Medical Association,* **251**, 630-632; 1984.

70. Rost, R. Physical exercise and antihypertensive drugs. *Nephron,* **47**(Suppl. 1):27-29; 1987.

71. Lund-Johansen, P. Exercise and antihypertensive therapy. *American Journal of Cardiology,* **59**, 98A-107A; 1987.

72. Georgopoulos, A.J., Proudfit, W.L., and Page, I.H. Effect of exercise on electrocardiogram of patients with low serum potassium. *Circulation,* **23**, 567-572; 1961.

73. Kaiser, P., Hylander, B., Eliasson, K., et al. Effect of beta$_1$-selective and nonselective beta blockade on blood pressure relative to physical performance in men with systemic hypertension. *American Journal of Cardiology,* **55**, 79D-84D; 1985.

74. Wilmore, J.H., Freund, B.J., Joyner, M.J., et al. Acute response to submaximal and maximal exercise consequent to beta-adrenergic blockade: implications for the prescription of exercise. *American Journal of Cardiology,* **55**, 135D-141D; 1985.

75. Hossack, K.F., Bruce, R.A., and Kusumi, F. Altered exercise ventilatory responses by apparent propranolol-diminished glucose metabolism: implications concerning impaired physical training benefit in coronary patients. *American Heart Journal,* **102**, 378-382; 1981.

76. Zohman, L.R. Exercise stress test interpretation for cardiac diagnosis and functional evaluation. *Archives of Physical Medicine and Rehabilitation,* **58**, 235-240; 1977.

77. Pratt, C.M., Welton, D.E., Squires, W.G., et al. Demonstration of training effect during chronic beta-adrenergic blockage in patients with coronary artery disease. *Circulation,* **64**, 1125-1129; 1981.

78. Froelicher, V., Sullivan, M., Myers, J., et al. Can patients with coronary artery disease receiving beta blockers obtain a training effect? *American Journal of Cardiology,* **55**, 155D-161D; 1985.
79. Vanhees, L., Fagard, R., and Amery, A. Influence of beta-adrenergic blockade on the hemodynamic effects of physical training in patients with ischemic heart disease. *American Heart Journal,* **108**, 270-275; 1984.
80. Hossack, K.F., Bruce, R.A., and Clark, L.J. Influence of propranolol on exercise prescription of training heart rates. *Cardiology,* **65**, 47-58; 1980.
81. Franklin, B.A., Gordon, S., and Timmis, G.C. Diurnal variation of ischemic response to exercise in patients receiving a once-daily dose of beta-blockers: implications for exercise testing and prescription of exercise and training heart rates. *Chest,* **109**, 253-257; 1996.
82. Fagard, R., Bulpitt, C., Lijnen, P., et al. Response of the systemic and pulmonary circulation to converting-enzyme inhibition (captopril) at rest and during exercise in hypertensive patients. *Circulation,* **65**, 33-39; 1982.
83. Mooy, J., van Baak, M., Bohm, R., et al. The effects of verapamil and propranolol on exercise tolerance in hypertensive patients. *Clinical Pharmacology and Therapeutics,* **41**, 490-495; 1987.
84. Myburgh, D.P., and Gordon, N.F. Comparison of diltiazem and atenolol in young, physically active men with essential hypertension. *American Journal of Cardiology,* **60**, 1092-1095; 1987.
85. Szlachcic, J., Hirsch, A.T., Tubau, J.F., et al. Diltiazem versus propranolol in essential hypertension: responses of rest and exercise blood pressure and effects on exercise capacity. *American Journal of Cardiology,* **59**, 393-399; 1987.
86. Chang, K., and Hossack, K.F. Effect of diltiazem on heart rate responses and respiratory variables during exercise: implications for exercise prescription and cardiac rehabilitation. *Journal of Cardiac Rehabilitation,* **2**, 326-332; 1982.
87. Sketch, M.H., Mooss, A.N., Butler, M.L., et al. Digoxin-induced positive exercise tests: their clinical and prognostic significance. *American Journal of Cardiology,* **48**, 655-659; 1981.
88. Schlant, R.C., Blomqvist, C.G., and Brandenburg, R.O., et al. Guidelines for exercise testing. *Circulation,* **74**, 653A-667A; 1986.
89. Van Camp, S.P., and Peterson, R.A. Cardiovascular complications of outpatient cardiac rehabilitation programs. *Journal of the American Medical Association,* **256**, 1160-1163; 1986.
90. Cobb, L.A., and Weaver, W.D. Exercise: a risk for sudden death in patients with coronary heart disease. *Journal of the American College of Cardiology,* **7**, 215-219; 1986.
91. Mittleman, M.A., Maclure, M., Tofler, G.H., et al. Triggering of acute myocardial infarction by heavy physical exertion: protection against triggering by regular exertion. *New England Journal of Medicine,* **329**, 1677-1683; 1993.
92. Willich, S.N., Lewis, M., Lowell, H., et al. Physical exertion as a trigger of acute myocardial infarction. *New England Journal of Medicine,* **329**, 1684-1690; 1993.
93. Mead, W.F., Pyfer, H.R., Trombold, J.C., et al. Successful resuscitation of two near simultaneous cases of cardiac arrest with a review of fifteen cases occurring during supervised exercise. *Circulation,* **53**, 187-189; 1976.

94. Hossack, K.F., and Hartwig, R. Cardiac arrest associated with supervised cardiac rehabilitation. *Journal of Cardiac Rehabilitation,* **2**, 402-408; 1982.

95. Friedwald, V.E., Jr., and Spence, D.W. Sudden cardiac death associated with exercise: the risk-benefit issue. *American Journal of Cardiology,* **66**, 183-188; 1990.

96. Thompson, P.D. The benefits and risks of exercise training in patients with coronary artery disease. *Journal of the American Medical Association,* **259**, 1537-1540; 1988.

97. Tran, Z.V., and Brammell, H.L. Effects of exercise training on serum lipid and lipoprotein levels in post-MI patients: a meta-analysis. *Journal of Cardiopulmonary Rehabilitation,* **9**, 250-255; 1989.

98. Sanne, H. Physical training after myocardial infarction. *Bibliography of Cardiology,* **36**, 164-173; 1976.

99. Hakkila, J. Morbidity and mortality after myocardial infarction. *Bibliography of Cardiology,* **36**, 159-163; 1976.

100. Kentala, E. Physical fitness and feasibility of physical rehabilitation after myocardial infarction in men of working age. *Annals of Clinical Research,* **4**(Suppl. 9):1-96; 1972.

101. Palatsi, I. Feasibility of physical training after myocardial infarction and its effects on return to work, morbidity and mortality. *Acta Medica Scandinavia,* **599**(Suppl.):7; 1976.

102. Kallio, V., Hamalainen, H., Hakkila, J., et al. Reduction in sudden deaths by a multifactorial intervention program after acute myocardial infarction. *Lancet,* **2**, 1091-1094; 1979.

103. Shaw, L.W. Effects of a prescribed exercise program on mortality and cardiovascular morbidity in patients after a myocardial infarction. *American Journal of Cardiology,* **48**, 36-49; 1981.

104. Shephard, R.J. Evaluation of earlier studies. The Canadian Study. In: Cohen, L.S., Mock, M.B., Ringqvist, I., eds. *Physical conditioning and cardiovascular rehabilitation.* New York: Wiley; 1981:pp. 271-287.

105. Roman, O., Gutierrez, M., Luksic, I., et al. Cardiac rehabilitation after acute myocardial infarction: nine-year controlled follow-up study. *Cardiology,* **70**, 223-231; 1983.

106. O'Connor, G.T., Buring, J.E., Yusuf, S., et al. An overview of randomized trials of rehabilitation with exercise after myocardial infarction. *Circulation,* **80**, 234-244; 1989.

107. Oldridge, N.B., Guyatt, G.H., Fisher, M.E., et al. Cardiac rehabilitation after myocardial infarction: combined experience of randomized clinical trials. *Journal of the American Medical Association,* **260**, 945-950; 1988.

108. Lau, J., Antman, E.M., Jimenez-Silva, J., et al. Cumulative meta-analysis of therapeutic trials for myocardial infarction. *New England Journal of Medicine,* **327**, 248-254; 1992.

109. American College of Sports Medicine Position Stand: exercise for patients with coronary artery disease. *Medicine and Science in Sports and Exercise,* **26**(3)i-v; 1994.

110. Blair, S.N., Kohl, H.W., Paffenbarger, R.S., et al. Physical fitness and all-cause mortality: a prospective study of healthy men and women. *Journal of the American Medical Association,* **262**, 2395-2401; 1989.

111. Blair, S.N., Kohl, H.W., Barlow, C.E., et al. Changes in physical fitness and all-cause mortality. A prospective study of healthy and unhealthy men. *Journal of the American Medical Association,* **273**, 1093-1098; 1995.

112. Franklin, B.A., Oldridge, N.B., Stoedefalke, K.G., et al. *On the ball: innovative activities for adult fitness and cardiac rehabilitation programs.* Carmel, IN: Benchmark Press; 1990.

113. Sotile, W.M. *Psychosocial interventions for cardiopulmonary patients.* Champaign, IL: Human Kinetics; 1996.

114. Ades, P.A., Waldmann, M.L., McCann, W.J., et al. Predictors of cardiac rehabilitation participation in older patients. *Archives of Internal Medicine,* **152**, 1033-1035; 1992.

115. Prochaska, J., and Di Clemente, C. Transtheoretical therapy, toward a more integrative model of change. *Psychiatric Theory and Research Practices,* **19**, 276-288; 1982.

116. Heinzelman, F., and Bagley, R.W. Response to physical activity programs and their effects on health behavior. *Public Health Reports,* **85**, 905-911; 1970.

Chapter 2

Resistive Exercise Training in Cardiac Rehabilitation

David E. Verrill, MS, FAACVPR

Introduction

Resistive exercise training has become very popular in cardiopulmonary rehabilitation programs (CRPs). Most people lack the physical strength and confidence to perform everyday activities effectively after a cardiac event, and it is vitally important for CRP participants of all ages to maintain or regain strength in order to return to daily vocational and recreational activities. Improvement in upper- and lower-body strength allows the CRP participant to perform everyday activities at a lower energy cost and with greater efficiency of movement. Patients who have jobs that require frequent lifting or frequent isometric contractions can prepare to resume those activities through resistive exercise (1-3). Resistive training has been shown to improve muscular strength, bone mass, cardiovascular endurance, self-image, and lean body mass (4-15). Conflicting data have been presented on the effect of resistive exercise on blood pressure, flexibility, and lipid/lipoprotein enhancement (4, 6, 7, 13). Further research is needed in these areas, especially in women.

Older cardiac patients are now encouraged to participate in resistive exercise. Many recent studies have shown that this form of training is highly effective for improving strength, balance, functional capacity, and bone density in geriatric populations. Greater lean body mass and bone mineral content may reduce the incidence of osteoporosis and complications associated with accidental falls in older patients (4, 13). Moreover, this form of training improves carbohydrate metabolism through lean body mass development, which has a positive effect on basal metabolism.

Nonsustained isometric or isodynamic activities, previously contraindicated for cardiac patients, are now recommended, since many vocations and everyday activities require frequent lifting/pushing movements that involve isometric muscle contractions (1, 16-18). The safety of repetitive weight lifting and carrying has been well documented in selected cardiac patients (19-27). Thus, it is now recommended that patients perform isodynamic arm and leg exercises during CRP sessions to help facilitate earlier return to work. These exercises should correspond with tasks performed during daily vocational and recreational activities (1-3, 17, 24, 27).

Many guidelines have been published on cardiac resistive exercise (17, 28-33). However, many questions remain unanswered. This chapter will analyze current research on resistive training to provide a framework for CRP staff and participants for safe and effective resistive exercise testing and training.

Physiologic Adaptations

In the past, resistive exercise training was regarded as hemodynamically unsafe for patients with coronary artery disease (CAD) and for the elderly. Weight lifting has been associated with a large increase in heart rate (HR) and/or blood pressure (BP) in healthy subjects (34, 35) and in those with CAD (36, 37). However, several studies have demonstrated that isotonic, isodynamic, and circuit weight training (CWT) programs using low, moderate, and even high levels of resistance are physiologically safe and effective for strength development in many cardiac populations (5, 8, 9, 36-45). Aerobically trained cardiac patients have shown significant gains in strength without cardiovascular complications following resistive training up to 80% of a 1 repetition maximum (1 RM) lift (5, 8, 41, 42). Resistive workloads of 50-80% of 1 RM have been shown to improve muscle size and strength, lean body mass, balance, bone mineral density, and endurance, and to be hemodynamically safe for older subjects up to 90 years of age (46-50). Further research is required to fully assess the cardiovascular risks, benefits, and complication rates of higher-intensity resistive exercise in older cardiac patients, special populations, and those with valvular disease or impaired left ventricular (LV) function. The following is a summary of the chronic physiologic adaptations that have been observed with resistive exercise in cardiac populations or those at risk of having a cardiac event (see also table 2.1):

- Enhanced self-efficacy, psychosocial well-being, (11, 12, 38) and higher patient confidence levels with strength-specific tasks (12)
- No change in body weight after up to 24 weeks of low- or high-intensity resistive training (8, 9, 41, 42)
- A small decrease in body fat in cardiac patients after 16 weeks of training (8) with no body fat changes observed in the same patients after 3 years of combined resistive and aerobic training (38)
- Lower resting and submaximal exercise HRs, increased resting and submaximal exercise stroke volume, and increased maximal exercise cardiac output in coronary artery bypass graft (CABG) patients after up to 12 weeks of CWT (5, 51)
- No change in systolic, diastolic, or mean BP in hypertensive men and women (10, 46, 52) or in cardiac patients (42) after up to 24 weeks of CWT
- A 4-15% increase in estimated or measured $\dot{V}O_2$max in low-risk cardiac patients after up to 16 weeks of exclusive CWT or CWT combined with aerobic exercise (5, 8, 9, 51, 53-55)
- A 20-40% increase in strength (5, 8, 9, 38, 42, 43)
- Conflicting data on whether resistive exercise favorably alters selected lipid or lipoprotein values in healthy or high-risk populations (6, 7, 10, 56-58)

- Improved glucose tolerance and enhanced insulin sensitivity in healthy subjects and in those with non-insulin-dependent diabetes mellitus (10, 59, 60).

At the present time, it appears that resistive and combined resistive/aerobic exercise increase strength, aerobic capacity, and cardiovascular function in cardiac populations. While resistive training also appears to enhance insulin sensitivity in healthy subjects or those at increased risk of cardiac event, it does not appear to enhance lipid values or lower BP.

Isometric and Isodynamic Exercise

Isometric exercise occurs repeatedly in daily activities and is the dominant form of exercise in many jobs as well. After a cardiac event, patients should be able to resume upper-body or isodynamic activities, such as carrying groceries, vacuuming, or pushing a lawn mower, as soon as possible. Because cardiac rehabilitation programs have traditionally focused on lower-body exercise, they may not have met the patient's individual vocational and avocational goals. Programs that incorporate isodynamic exercise (e.g., walking with elastic bands, carrying weights) may prepare the patient to resume daily upper-body activities and improve quality of life better than those that do not feature such exercise. Important benefits of upper-body resistive training include the reduction of dyspnea with daily isodynamic activities, improvement of respiratory muscle function, and an increase in work tolerance.

Isometric work (weight lifting, squeezing, or pressing) involves constant muscle contraction of a muscle group and is primarily anaerobic, since muscle blood flow and oxygen delivery are compromised with sustained compression of arterial vessels during contraction. (61-64) Clinical investigators have reported that during sustained isometric exercise, patients with mild to severe LV impairment or congestive heart failure may demonstrate

- a decrease in cardiac output, stroke volume, and ejection fraction,
- an increase in LV end-diastolic pressure,
- regional wall motion abnormalities,
- mitral regurgitation, and
- dysrhythmias (1, 18, 66-69).

Thus, sustained or high-intensity isometric exercise has been regarded as unsafe for patients with poor LV function because of the excessive level of myocardial pressure work and has traditionally been contraindicated for all cardiac patients because of the adverse effects of increased afterload and associated ischemia (61, 70).

Many studies have shown that handgrip or weighted exercise alone, or in combination with dynamic exercise, produces less ischemic ST-segment depression and arrhythmias than graded exercise testing (25, 69-73). Investigations using isometric or isodynamic exercise (i.e., weight-loaded walking, weight carrying and lifting, or vocational work simulation) have not shown adverse cardiac responses such as angina, significant ST-segment depression, or significant dysrhythmias in patients who

Table 2.1   A Summary of 12 Circuit Weight Training Studies in Male Cardiac Patients

Study	N	Clinical status	Duration of training	Mode/intensity of CWT	Strength gains	Aerobic capacity	Cardiovascular complications	% Fat/ weight change
Haennel et al., 1991	8	CABG (9-10 weeks post surg.)	8 weeks	3 circuits, 8-16 reps, 20 sec work intervals	22% incr. in upper, 18% incr. in lower body strength	11% incr. in VO_2max	None	No changes
Squires et al., 1991	13	MI, CABG (4 pts. EF < 40%, 5-6 weeks post-event)	Averaged 6 weight-lifting sessions	1 circuit, 10-14 reps. of a 10 rep. RM estimate; aerobic exercise	25% ave. increase in upper/lower body/strength	Not measured	None	Not reported
Sparling et al., 1990	16	PTCA, CABG MI, CAD, "high risk"	24 weeks, 3×/week	1 circuit at 30-40% of 1 RM; aerobic exercise 70-85% of HRmax	22% ave. incr. in upper/lower body strength	Not measured	None	No changes
McCartney et al., 1991	10	CAD, MI, CABG, angina	10 weeks, 2×/week	2 circuits at 40-80% of 1 RM; aerobic exercise 60-85% of HRmax	42% incr. in upper, 23% incr. in lower body strength	15% incr. in max cycle power output; 109% incr. in max cycle time	None	Not reported
Ghilarducci et al., 1989	9	MI, angina, CABG	10 weeks, 3×/week	1 circuit at 80% of 1 RM; sit-ups; aerobic exercise at 45-64% of HRmax	29% ave. incr. in upper/lower body strength	Not measured	None	No changes
Kelemen et al., 1986	20	MI, CAD, CABG, angina	10 weeks, 3×/week	2 circuits at 40% of 1 RM; aerobic exercise at 85% of HRmax	24% ave. incr. in upper/lower body strength	12% incr. in Bruce treadmill time	1 pt. hypotensive; 4 pts. PVCs with bigeminy	No weight change; small decrease in body fat

Study	N	Population	Duration/frequency	Training protocol	Strength	Aerobic capacity		
Svedahl et al., 1994	16	8-12 weeks post-MI (ave. EF = 40-45%)	12 weeks, 3×/week	Hydraulic CWT, 40 min/day, 3 days/week, 20-sec. work: rest intervals	29% incr. upper, 23% incr. in lower body strength	19% incr. in $\dot{V}O_2$max; 23% incr. in peak cycle ergometer workload	None	Not reported
Stewart et al., 1994	8	≥2 weeks post-MI (no anterior Q wave)	10 weeks, 3×/week	2 circuits at 40% of 1 RM; aerobic exercise	22% incr. upper, 29% incr. in lower body strength	15% incr. in $\dot{V}O_2$max	None	No changes
Wilke et al., 1991	14	MI, CABG, PTCA, angina, valvular	12 weeks, 3×/week	3 circuits at 40-70% of 1 RM; aerobic exercise at 70-85% of HRmax	30% incr. upper, 35% incr. in lower body strength	14% incr. in $\dot{V}O_2$max	None	Not reported
Stewart et al., 1988	17	MI, CAD, CABG (follow-up of Kelemen et al., 1986)	3 years, 3×/week	2 circuits at 40% of 1 RM; aerobic exercise at 85% of HRmax	13% incr. upper, 40% incr. in lower body strength	Not measured	None	No changes
Derman et al., 1994	9	CRP participants	10 weeks	CWT (intensity not specified); aerobic exercise	19% incr. in max. isometric voluntary contraction	No change in $\dot{V}O_2$max; 19% incr. in cycle time to exhaustion	None	Not reported
Daub et al., 1996	57	6-16 weeks post-MI	10 weeks	2 circuits at 20-60% of 1 RM; aerobic exer. at 70-85% HRmax	10.5-13.5% incr. in upper body strength	4.4-13.4% incr. in $\dot{V}O_2$max	None	Not reported

Reprinted with permission from D.E. Verrill and P.M. Ribisl, 1996, "Resistive exercise training in cardiac rehabilitation—an update," *Sports Medicine* 21(5):362.
Abbreviations: CABG = Coronary artery bypass grafting; MI = Myocardial infarction; EF = Ejection fraction; CAD = Coronary artery disease; PTCA = Percutaneous transluminal coronary angioplasty; 1RM = One repetition maximum; $\dot{V}O_2$max = Maximal oxygen uptake; HR = heart rate; PVC = Premature ventricular contraction; pt(s) = patient(s); incr. = increase; ave. = average; and CRP = Cardiopulmonary rehabilitation program.

have had CABG or uncomplicated myocardial infarction (MI) (2, 19-27, 72-75). Moreover, some feel that isometric/isodynamic exercise may actually favor myocardial perfusion at rate-pressure products (RPPs) that normally produce ischemic ECG changes during dynamic exercise (18, 69, 71). This is the case because the elevated diastolic BP and decreased venous return and wall tension observed during isometric exercise (61, 64) may actually increase coronary perfusion pressure and improve coronary blood flow to collaterals and stenotic areas during diastole, thereby reducing the development of myocardial ischemia (17, 40, 41, 69, 72). Thus, including nonsustained isometric and isodynamic exercises in medically supervised programs may better prepare your patients for faster return to occupational and leisure activities. Figure 2.1 a and b illustrates an isodynamic elastic band activity that one can perform while walking.

Individualized exercise prescriptions for low-intensity isometric/isodynamic exercise should consider the patient's cardiovascular status (e.g., LV function), long-term goals, and occupational requirements (1, 18, 62). Various isometric tests such as handgrip dynamometer, elastic tube, or dead-lift testing may be useful in this respect. Monitored exercise tests that involve weight lifting or carrying for work simulation may also be used to accurately prescribe vocational or avocational activities (76). While isometric/isodynamic testing has generally been shown to be hemodynamically safe in cardiac populations, some investigators have observed frequent premature ventricular contractions (PVCs), elevated diastolic BPs, and/or marked fluctuations in BP during weight-lifting/weight-carrying tasks in some patients (8, 75). You should always warn patients against breath-holding or prolonged isometric contractions and caution them to avoid daily activities that may involve heavy lifting or pushing (e.g., shoveling wet snow, pushing a car, carrying a heavy suitcase, splitting hardwood) (77-79). It is very important that they are aware of the dangers of the Valsalva maneuver.

Resistance-Training Equipment

A wide variety of resistance-training equipment is currently being used in CRPs for strength development and improvement. This list continues to grow daily as new, less expensive devices reach the market. Resistive modalities range from weighted bags to expensive machines. Table 2.2 presents a summary of the advantages and disadvantages of some of these devices. Many types of equipment lend themselves to gradual progression of resistance. Inpatient (phase I) participants should use light resistive equipment (e.g., light dumbbells, squeeze balls, low-tension elastic bands) and/or light resistive calisthenics to help regain strength after an acute cardiac event. Participants in phase II programs are generally advised to use lighter levels of resistance during the early sessions to avoid potential joint injury, orthopedic complications, or sternotomy complications after surgery (80). Machines, free weights, hand/wrist/ankle weights, walking poles, and elastic bands/tubes are just some of the resistive devices currently being used for muscle conditioning in phase II-III programs. In the following sections each modality will be discussed separately.

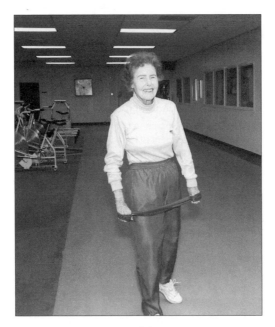

1a

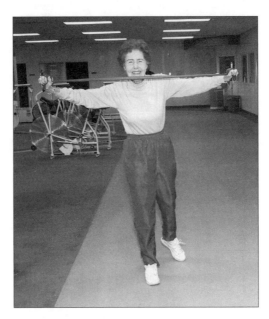

1b

Figure 2.1a and b   Exercise with elastic bands offers an isodynamic activity that a patient can perform while walking.

Table 2.2   Types of Resistance-Training Equipment

	Advantages	Disadvantages
Cuff, hand, and ankle weights	• Minimal storage and exercise space • Easily moved, lightweight • Large number of patients may participate simultaneously • No isometric component with wrist or ankle wraps •Increased energy cost of activity • Cost effective	• Possible adverse hemodynamic response in selected patients with hand gripping • Potential for connective tissue damage with excessive arm swinging • Potential for leg/hip injury when running with ankle weights
Dumbbells	• Minimal storage and exercise space • Easily moved • Isolate specific muscles better than other modalities • Large number of patients may participate simultaneously • Gradual progression of resistance • Cost effective	• Possible adverse hemodynamic response for selected patients • Isometric component with hand gripping • Weights may be dropped
Bands/tubes	• Minimal storage and exercise space • Easily moved • Gradual progression of resistance • Distribute resistive force, preventing impaired circulation • Large number of patients may participate simultaneously • Potential for increased joint flexibility • Cost effective	• Possible adverse hemodynamic response for selected patients • Isometric component with sustained pulling of bands/tubes • Resistance is lowest at the beginning and highest at the end of muscle contraction • Tear easily with sharp objects (e.g., rings, bracelets)
Walking poles	• Increased metabolic cost of walking • Safe, low isometric component • Large number of patients may participate simultaneously • Cost effective	• Can only be used while walking
Barbells	• Gradual progression of resistance • Greater potential for improvements in strength • Isolate specific muscles better than other modalities	• "Spotters" may be necessary • Increased skill level required • Isometric component • Weights may be dropped • Usually heavier resistance due to weight of bar
Machine weights	• Large selection of equipment available • Reduced isometric component • No "spotters" necessary • Easily determined and precise weight exercise prescription	• Large space requirement • Small number of patients may participate simultaneously • Increased cost of equipment • Moving equipment from site to site difficult

cont.

Table 2.2   (continued)

	Advantages	Disadvantages
	• Enjoyable and motivational—increases exercise compliance • Multistation machines available for increased patient participation	
Circuit weight training	• Possible to incorporate any of the aforementioned components into a circuit—offers flexibility and variety • Machine weights most popular due to safety and absence of "spotters" • Potential for increased strength, aerobic capacity, favorable body composition changes, and risk factor reduction • More time efficient—able to incorporate more resistive exercise into rehab session • Enjoyable—greater exercise compliance	• Large space requirement • Potential for minimal number of patients to participate simultaneously due to time and space allotment • Increased cost of equipment if machines are used

Adapted from D.E. Verrill and P.M. Ribisl, 1996, "Resistive exercise training in cardiac rehabilitation—an update," *Sports Medicine* 21(5):365.

Machine Weights

Isotonic, isokinetic, or hydraulic machines (e.g., Cybex, Nautilus, Universal), if affordable, can provide patients the opportunity to improve both muscular strength and cardiovascular endurance. Most are used in a single- or multi-station format. Machines are enjoyable, easy to learn, and may contribute to greater exercise compliance. A number of new machines on the market are space efficient and provide for a wide variety of muscular strengthening exercises. While some of the higher-grade machines are expensive and cost prohibitive for CRPs, many newer models are lighter, less expensive, and sturdy enough for daily use in a rehabilitation program. Machines have the advantage of protecting the back by stabilizing the patient's body position and allowing the workload to be increased by small increments. Some machines are equipped with range-of-motion limitation for patients with orthopedic problems. From a safety standpoint, light machine weights are preferable to barbells for geriatric patients. If patients purchase weight machines for home use, it is imperative they have instruction on the safety, function, durability, and maintenance of the machine. Many of the newer devices seen in infomercials are not sturdy enough for daily use. Thus, before patients purchase home equipment, they should talk to the CRP exercise specialist, physical therapist, or athletic trainer.

Free Weights

Free weights (barbells and dumbbells) can and should be used in CRPs, provided proper technique is emphasized. Light dumbbells (1-15 lb) come in varying colors for different weights and can be used in a variety of exercises for upper-body strength development (see fig. 2.2). Heavier dumbbells or barbells may not be suitable for older patients who might drop them or use them ineffectively; they also may cause patients with balance problems to fall. Low-level machine exercise or elastic exercise is more suitable than free weights for those with neuromuscular impairment or balance problems. Heavier free weights (e.g., dumbbells and barbells weighing 25 lb or more) should be used only for stronger patients with higher functional capacities. Staff spotters may be necessary for those who have progressed to heavier workloads.

Walking Poles

Walking poles are ski pole-like devices with rubber tips that can be used to enhance upper-body strength and muscular endurance for patients during indoor or outdoor track walking. The patient uses the poles while walking as one would use poles during cross-country skiing. The poles are effective in that they do not promote an exces-

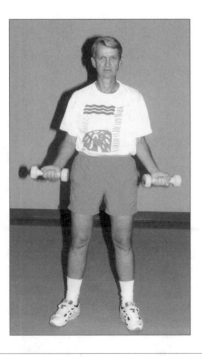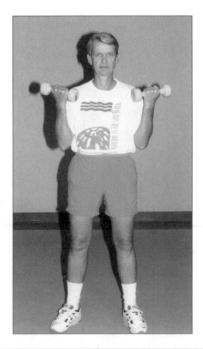

Figure 2.2   Light dumbbells can be used in a variety of exercises for upper-body strength.

sive pressor response; there is a supportive strap, located near the wrist, that reduces the need to grip the pole itself. Walking poles have been shown to increase HR by 14 beats $\cdot$ min^{-1} (68% to 78% of HRmax) and $\dot{V}O_2$ by 3.8 ml $\cdot$ kg^{-1} $\cdot$ min^{-1} (21%) as compared to values for walking without poles in male patients with previous CABG or MI (81). The patients should have individualized instruction and practice sessions so that they become familiar with proper walking technique. Walking poles are inexpensive and are excellent for increasing energy expenditure and muscular endurance for those patients who perform walking as a primary activity during CRP sessions.

Handheld, Cuff, and Ankle Weights

Handheld, cuff, and ankle weights may be used during floor exercise or in conjunction with aerobic activities in CRPs. These weights generally range from 0.45 to 11.4 kg (1-25 lb) and are portable and inexpensive. Walking with handheld or wrist weights is isodynamic and may increase metabolic and hemodynamic exercise responses. Thus this equipment may provide some cardiovascular benefit for the cardiac participant. However, these modalities have been criticized because of the potential for joint injury or orthopedic complications with improper use in untrained patients or in patients with musculoskeletal limitations. Using handheld weights during walking has been regarded as unsafe for hypertensive individuals because of the potential for high BP elevations from increased peripheral resistance and muscle tension with isometric gripping (82-86). Investigations with hypertensive responders (84), healthy subjects (82), older men and women (mean age 66.2 $\pm$ 5.6 years) (85), and cardiac patients (86) all have shown exaggerated BP responses as high as 250/110 mm Hg with hand-weighted walking in some subjects. In cardiac populations, gripping handheld weights could potentially increase HR and systolic BP through the pressor response, increasing the RPP and myocardial oxygen demand. This could be dangerous if patients exercise beyond their ischemic threshold. Conversely, the ischemic threshold may be improved with combined static and dynamic exercise in patients with CAD. Moreover, the increase in diastolic BP reported in many of these studies with weighted walking may improve coronary perfusion and myocardial oxygen supply in CRP participants. Thus, this topic remains controversial.

In apparently healthy subjects, the physiologic responses with use of light (0.45-2.27 kg or 1-5 lb) cuff or hand weights are generally mild (82-84, 87-91). These responses include

- a small increase in the metabolic cost of walking (overall increase of 1.2-3.8 ml $\cdot$ kg^{-1} $\cdot$ min^{-1});
- no change or a small increase in HR (4-13 beats $\cdot$ min^{-1});
- no change or a small increase in rating of perceived exertion (RPE), generally 0-2 units on the Borg category scale;
- no change or a small increase in systolic BP (12-18 mm Hg) with a wide variation in hypertensive responders;
- a mild to moderate increase in diastolic BP (2-10 mm Hg); and
- a mild increase in RPP (20-38 mm Hg $\cdot$ min^{-1}).

Greater metabolic and hemodynamic responses have been reported in older subjects (85) with heavier weights, and with exaggerated arm swings in younger subjects (87-89). The reported variations among studies are due to differences in weight load, degree of arm swing, stride length, work intensity, subject fitness level, subject age, time of HR/BP measurement, and/or the degree of isometric contraction with hand gripping.

Generally no change, or only mild physiologic changes, have been observed in low-risk cardiac patients during weighted walking. Amos et al. (86) observed a mild increase in HR and BP with no ischemic ECG responses during treadmill walking using 1.14 kg (2.5 lb) ankle or wrist weights in patients with CAD. In this investigation, wrist weights generally elicited greater hemodynamic responses than ankle weights. One subject had an exaggerated BP response of 230/120 mm Hg during weighted walking and was not allowed to finish the trial. Landi et al. (74) observed that cardiac patients who carried 4 kg (8.8 lb) weights with elbows flexed had a greater rise in systolic BP (154 ± 16 mm Hg) than those who carried weights with elbows extended (142 ± 13 mm Hg).

There has been little research on musculoskeletal complications or physiologic adaptations associated with wrist or ankle weight-loaded walking in cardiac populations. Vigorous arm/leg movements or running during weighted exercise could put excessive pressure on the shoulder, elbow, or ankle joints and may result in connective tissue damage. Furthermore, hypertensive patients could exacerbate BP with hand-weight gripping during extended track or treadmill walking. It is recommended that patients with hypertension or a history of musculoskeletal injuries be thoroughly screened before participation in weighted exercise. If patients are using hand or ankle weights, they should avoid exaggerated arm swings or stride patterns in order to protect joints. Patients should not jog or run with hand, wrist, or ankle weights because of the potential for joint stress or adverse hemodynamic effects. Monitored exercise tests on patients with attached cuffs or on those holding weights may provide useful information regarding the cardiovascular and/or musculoskeletal responses during weighted exercise. With this form of testing, you can more accurately prescribe exercise for patients who wish to participate in weighted exercise and identify those patients who exhibit exaggerated HR or BP responses.

Patient Screening and Contraindications

Although cardiovascular complications have been shown to be rare with resistive training, this form of exercise may pose a hazard to higher-risk patients who are predisposed to adverse cardiac events. Therefore, it is important to properly screen all individuals for participation in resistive exercise. Generally, patients should not participate in resistive exercise if they have

- an abnormal hemodynamic response or significant ischemic ECG changes during graded exercise;
- poor LV function (ejection fraction <30%);

Contraindications for Participation in Resistive Exercise Training[1]

Absolute Contraindications

1. Resting, changing pattern, or new onset of angina pectoris

2. Complex supraventricular or ventricular dysrhythmias at rest or dysrhythmias that worsen with exercise

3. Uncompensated or symptomatic congestive heart failure

4. Recent MI, chest surgery, or episode of cardiac arrest (<2 weeks)

5. Multiple or complicated MIs

6. Severe or symptomatic aortic stenosis

7. Severely depressed LV function (ejection fraction <30%)

8. Severe CAD (high left anterior descending, triple vessel)

9. Exertional hypotension ($\geq$ 15 mm Hg) or failure of BP to rise during graded exercise

10. A recent change in the resting ECG suggesting infarction or other acute cardiac event

11. Significant exercise-induced ST-segment depression ($\geq$ 3 mm flat or downsloping)

12. Recent complicated MI or recurrent/persistent ischemic symptoms post-cardiac event

13. History of large, unrepaired cerebral, thoracic, abdominal, or ventricular aneurysm

14. Active or suspected myocarditis, pericarditis, or endocarditis

15. Thrombophlebitis or intracardiac thrombi

16. Hypertrophic cardiomyopathy

17. Acute pulmonary embolus or pulmonary infarction

18. Third-degree or advanced atrioventricular block

19. Resting systolic BP > 200 mmHg and/or resting diastolic BP > 105 mm Hg

20. Any medical problem that warrants contraindication

21. Orthopedic problems that would prohibit resistive exercise

22. Uncontrolled metabolic disease (i.e., diabetes mellitus, myxedema, thyrotoxicosis)

23. Severe restrictive or obstructive lung disease

24. Acute episodes of joint inflammatory or degenerative disease (bursitis, arthritis, gout)

25. Advanced or complicated pregnancy

Relative Contraindications

1. Excessive BP rise with resistive exercise: systolic pressure $\geq$ 220 mm Hg or diastolic pressure $\geq$ 110 mm Hg

2. Frequent or complex ventricular ectopy

3. Congenital heart disease or congenital heart defects

4. Ischemic cardiomyopathy

5. Neuromuscular, musculoskeletal, or rheumatoid disorders exacerbated by exercise

6. Moderate valvular heart disease

7. Low exercise capacity (<3 METs)

8. Failure to comply with the resistive exercise prescription

9. Recent survivor of cardiac arrest

10. Chronic infectious disease (e.g., mononucleosis, AIDS, hepatitis)

11. Resting systolic BP $\geq$ 180 mm Hg and/or resting diastolic BP $\geq$ 100 mm Hg

[1]Adapted from AACVPR (28), ACSM (31), and AHA (92).

- a low functional capacity (≤3 METs);
- uncontrolled angina, heart failure, hypertension, or dysrhythmias;
- severe CAD (left main, triple-vessel, or high left anterior descending disease);
- severe or symptomatic aortic stenosis;
- clinically limiting orthopedic or cardiovascular symptomatology; or
- characteristics associated with an increased risk for cardiac events during exercise (8, 28, 31, 32, 39, 92).

Cardiopulmonary rehabilitation staff should consider patients who fall under the American College of Sports Medicine/American College of Physicians (ACSM/ACP) (31), American Association of Cardiovascular and Pulmonary Rehabilitation (AACVPR) (28), and/or American Heart Association (AHA) (92) high-risk stratification criteria as unsuitable candidates for participation in higher-intensity resistive exercise. An adaptation of these criteria that is specific to resistive exercise is presented on pages 53–54. Staff should also consider the contraindications for exercise testing and/or entry into cardiac exercise programs published by the ACSM (31) and AHA (92) as contraindications for patient participation in resistive exercise. Low- to moderate-risk patients may be well suited for resistive training and should be encouraged to participate. Low-level resistive exercise (e.g., low-tension bands, light dumbbells, walking poles) may be suitable for higher-risk patients or for the patient with a low functional capacity.

No serious cardiovascular complications associated with acute resistive training have been reported in the literature. Investigators who have compared cardiovascular responses during low-, moderate-, and even high-intensity weight lifting have universally reported fewer cardiac arrhythmias or ischemic signs/symptoms during weight lifting than during graded exercise. However, episodes of symptomatic hypotension (8), nonsymptomatic hypotension or wide BP fluctuation (24), and frequent PVCs or ventricular bigeminy (8, 22, 24, 26, 44) have been reported in some patients during or immediately following weight lifting or weight-loaded walking (i.e., walking with hand weights, ankle weights, or backpacks). Moreover, diastolic BPs appear to be significantly higher during weight lifting, weight carrying, or weight-loaded walking than during graded exercise (26, 36, 37, 40, 93, 94). All patients, especially those with a history of hypertension or hypotensive/syncopal episodes, should be screened carefully and instructed on safety precautions before resistive exercise participation. Most should have a functional capacity $\geq$ 6-7 METs (1 MET = 3.5 ml $\cdot$ kg^{-1} $\cdot$ min^{-1}) assessed from a symptom-limited graded exercise test prior to participation in higher-intensity resistive exercise (8, 30-32, 39). Low- to moderate-risk patients with functional capacities ≤6 METs may be able to safely perform resistive exercise in a circuit fashion with lighter workloads.

Resistive Training in High-Risk Populations

Should patients considered to be at a higher risk of cardiovascular complications (e.g., cardiomyopathy, impaired LV function) participate in resistive exercise? This area is controversial, and few studies have looked specifically at higher-risk patients. Dossa et al. (95) concluded that low-intensity strength training is well tolerated in elderly patients with ischemic cardiomyopathy and congestive heart failure, although further research is needed in other high-risk patient populations. Sheldahl et al. (24), Squires et al. (43), and Vander et al. (45) have all included higher-risk patients with low ejection fractions (12-40%) in their investigations and have observed no significant cardiovascular complications with moderate to high levels of resistive exercise testing and training. Sheldahl et al. (24) did report PVCs, elevated diastolic BPs, and angina in some subjects. Thus, it may be feasible to develop resistive-training regimens for some properly screened higher-risk CRP participants. However, since patients with low ejection fractions (i.e., <30%), cardiomyopathy, and severe valve disease or CAD are considered to be at high risk for complications, much additional study is needed in this area before you can routinely recommend resistive exercise for higher-risk patients.

Older patients are strongly encouraged to perform resistive training because of the potential for enhanced strength, bone mass, and cardiovascular function (4, 46-49). Strength training is also imperative in the cardiac transplant patient to counteract the effects of prednisone therapy, to improve daily function, and to enhance joint-loading capacity. A deficiency in leg strength has been shown to persist for up to 18 months after cardiac transplantation, perhaps contributing to lower peak oxygen consumption values observed in transplanted patients (96). Gradual progression of low resistive workloads with higher repetitions will help to develop strength in these patients (97). Low-level calisthenics and dynamic weight-bearing activities should also be incorporated in the resistive-training regimen. Isometric exercise is not recommended for transplanted patients because of the potential for an exaggerated BP response, which may already be elevated.

Resistive training may benefit CRP participants with other pathologic conditions. Those with mitral valve prolapse syndrome are encouraged to perform resistive exercise, but should avoid heavy weight lifting (98). Patients with peripheral arterial disease may see additional gains in strength after a resistive program, but may not improve peak oxygen consumption or onset time to leg claudication pain (99). Further research is needed in renal, cancer, and pulmonary patients to determine the benefits and safety of resistive exercise in these populations. It is ultimately the responsibility of the CRP staff to screen patients for participation in resistive exercise. Other contraindications for patient participation may exist and should be discussed on an individual basis. Current research strongly supports widespread participation in some form of resistive training for most CRP participants.

Exercise Prescription

You can implement a resistive exercise prescription for a cardiac patient using a creative format of exercises designed to strengthen all major muscle groups, especially those in the upper body. Many activities of daily living require more arm work than leg work, and patients should be prepared to resume upper-body activities as soon as possible after a cardiac event. The muscles of the lower body should also be strengthened to enhance lower-body strength, muscle mass, bone density, and to prevent musculoskeletal problems from occurring, such as low-back pain. Many combinations of modalities (e.g., weighted bags, hand weights, bands, machines) can be assembled in a separate training area with instructions and diagrams placed above each modality to show how to perform the specific exercise.

When to Begin Resistive Training

There is currently debate on how soon patients should begin resistive training after CRP entry. After hospital discharge and a medical evaluation that includes a symptom-limited graded exercise test, resistive exercise training should be initiated with the patient's cardiovascular status and functional capacity taken into account (28, 31, 80, 100). It has been recommended that patients participate regularly in CRP sessions for at least 12-16 weeks before beginning heavier resistive exercise (8, 30, 32). This period allows for sufficient clinical observation, patient education, and wound healing from CABG or other types of cardiac surgery. This also allows time for cardiorespiratory and musculoskeletal adaptations to occur. However, some investigators have shown that heavier weight lifting or CWT may be initiated as early as 2 to 10 weeks after MI or CABG surgery in properly screened, low- to moderate-risk patients (5, 43, 53-55, 94). Haennel et al. (5) observed that male patients 9-10 weeks post-CABG surgery who performed hydraulic CWT (three circuits per day, 12-16 repetitions per station) had no abnormal cardiovascular or musculoskeletal complications during resistive exercise testing or training. Stewart et al. (53) found that properly screened, low-risk male patients 2 weeks or more post-MI tolerated low-level CWT very well (12-15 repetitions at 40% of 1 RM) without sustained arrhythmias or ischemic episodes. They concluded that CWT may be incorporated into CRP sessions soon after MI to promote greater increases in strength and cardiovascular endurance than seen with aerobic exercise alone. Similarly, Daub et al. (55) found that low-risk male patients 6-16 weeks post-MI could participate in CWT without cardiac complications at workloads ranging from 20% to 60% of 1 RM. Squires et al. (43) also concluded that low risk male participants (mean age 45 ± 15 years) could safely perform machine resistive exercise early (≥17 days) after CABG surgery or MI. The ejection fractions of the subjects in this study ranged from 21% to 83% (mean ejection fraction = 48%), and four subjects had ejection fractions of less than 40%. No abnormal cardiovascular responses or sternotomy complications were noted during resistive testing or training in this patient population.

These findings suggest that heavier resistive exercise and CWT may be safely performed relatively early after a cardiac event for carefully screened, low- to moderate-risk patients. The AACVPR (28) recommends that CABG or MI patients perform 3-6 weeks of supervised aerobic exercise before beginning resistive exercise. The ACSM has similar recommendations for CABG and MI patients (4-6 weeks), but states that those with percutaneous transluminal coronary angioplasty or other revascularization procedures need wait only 1-2 weeks before beginning resistive training. The patient's cardiovascular status should dictate how soon he/she begins resistive training, and some patients may not be able to perform machine weights or CWT early after a cardiac event. Since neither the ACSM or AACVPR defines the recommended *level* of resistive exercise (e.g., light hand weights or machine weights at 60% of 1 RM), it is best to look at each patient on an individual basis to assess how soon he/she can begin resistive training and at what level.

Exercise Mode

Many resistive devices are available for use in CRPs, some of which were described earlier in this chapter (see section on resistance-training equipment). Isometric devices generate force without a change in muscle length and include handgrip dynamometers and sponge-type squeeze balls. Isotonic devices are dynamic in nature and generate force while the length of the muscle shortens (concentric contraction) or lengthens (eccentric contraction). These devices may generate force against a constant resistance (dumbbells, barbells, weighted bags) or a variable resistance (machines, wall pulleys). Isokinetic or accommodating resistance exercise involves dynamic exercise on devices that use exertion of force at a constant speed. These types of machines are best suited for athletes requiring training for specific dynamic movements during sports, and may be too expensive for many CRPs.

Once equipment has been purchased for your CRP, resistive exercise should be performed by patients slowly through the maximum range of motion that does not elicit pain or discomfort (31, 100–102). Patients who have had recent chest surgery should avoid exercises that put undue pressure on the sternum (e.g., heavy bench presses, "fly" movements). One must also use caution in prescribing above-the-shoulder arm exercises (e.g., military press) for patients with poor or unknown LV function because of the potential for generating high BP responses. Elderly patients may have limitations in neuromuscular coordination that may be exacerbated by fatigue; in this case, light machine weights or elastics may be preferable to free weights (see figs. 2.3 and 2.4).

All patients should perform abdominal strengthening exercises, either on mats or with machines. Many safe, effective, and biomechanically correct abdominal exercise devices are now commercially available at a low cost for the CRP ($40-$150). These types of exercises may benefit the patient through the development of better posture and prevention of low-back pain (see fig. 2.5).

Elastic exercise is excellent for phase II patients who have had recent CABG or other types of chest surgery because of its low level, graduated resistance, and the potential for range-of-motion improvement (see figs. 2.6 and 2.7). Elastic bands range in tension from very light to very hard and can be combined to increase resistance.

Various calisthenics that use rhythmic, dynamic movements of large muscle groups may be performed with or without resistive devices to supplement overall strength improvement. Aerobic equipment (e.g., wind-resistance cycle ergometers, rowing machines, isokinetic arm crank ergometers) can provide additional strength gains through arm, leg, or combined arm/leg exercise. Participants should always be monitored closely for proper form, abnormal symptoms, and signs of intolerance once they have begun resistive training on each piece of equipment or with other resistive modalities.

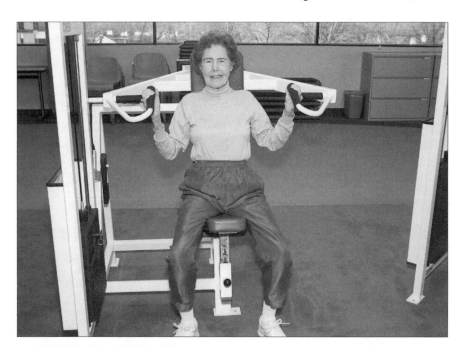

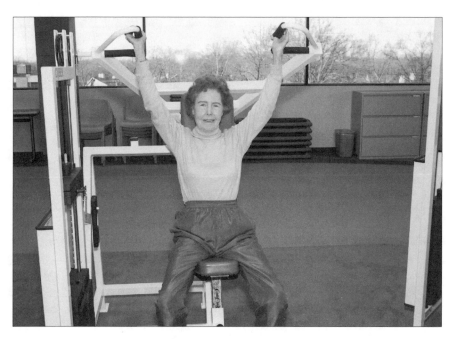

Figure 2.3   Light machine weights may be preferable to free weights for older patients.

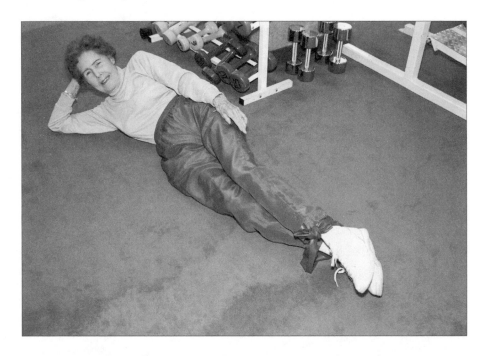

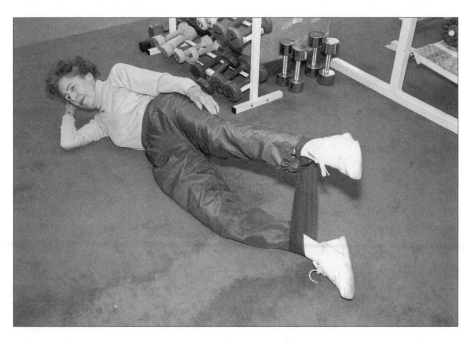

Figure 2.4 Elastics are preferable to free weights for some older patients.

Intensity

Initially, CRP participants should use the lightest resistance possible that can be lifted comfortably (17, 28, 32, 33). This normally corresponds to a workload of 30-50% of 1 RM or a weight that can be lifted for 8-10 repetitions comfortably. Whereas recent studies have shown that heavier resistive exercise (up to 100% of 1 RM) appears to be hemodynamically safe for some cardiac patients (5, 36, 40, 41, 44), it is more prudent for CRP personnel to use lower training workloads. Resistive exercise HRs should not exceed the prescribed aerobic target HRs and may often fall below target range, since resistive exercise appears to produce an increase in RPP through elevation of systolic BP with less contribution of HR. Thus, the RPP may be a better indicator of cardiovascular stress during exercise, and patients should not exceed an RPP at which signs or symptoms of myocardial ischemia appear during graded exercise (28, 33). The RPE should typically range from 11 to 14 ("light" to "somewhat hard") on the Borg category scale and from 3 to 6 ("moderate" to "more difficult") on the category-ratio scale during the resistive session.

The AACVPR (28) has recommended that low-risk cardiac patients initially perform resistive exercise at workloads corresponding to 30-50% of 1 RM. Although the addition of more sets, repetitions, resistance, or days of training may further enhance strength development, such gains appear to be relatively small. Heavy or highly repetitive resistive training that may increase the hemodynamic response and cardio-

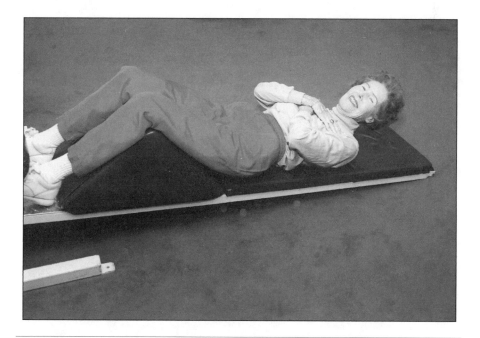

Figure 2.5   Performing abdominal strengthening exercises can help a patient develop better posture and prevent low-back pain.

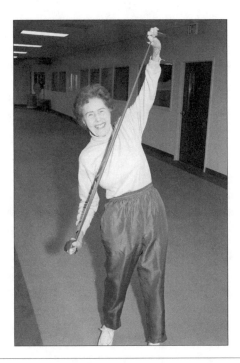

Figure 2.6   Elastic band exercise for the deltoid, triceps, and infraspinatus muscle groups.

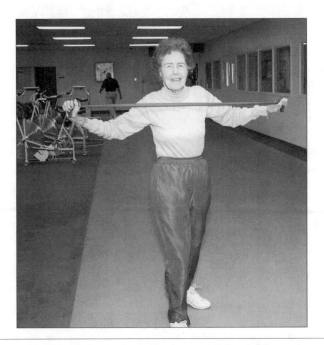

Figure 2.7   Elastic band exercise for the infraspinatus and rhomboid muscle groups.

vascular risk of resistive exercise, cause excessive fatigue, or increase musculoskeletal injuries offers little additional benefit in strength for the cardiac participant and may result in lower patient adherence (17, 44). Interestingly, Daub et al. (55) found *lower* increases in $\dot{V}O_2$max in post-MI patients with heavier CWT resistance levels (i.e., a 4.4% increase in $\dot{V}O_2$max with 60% of 1 RM training vs. 11.4% increase in $\dot{V}O_2$max with 20% of 1 RM training). Thus, lighter resistive training may overall be more beneficial to the patient than heavier, more difficult resistive training.

Number of Repetitions

In previous studies of cardiac patients, 10-15 repetitions of each exercise at 40-80% of 1 RM has been most often recommended for strength development. Initially, your patient should lift a light resistance for 8-12 repetitions. Over time, the workload may be increased up to 15 repetitions. Muscular strength is best developed with higher resistance, and muscular endurance is best developed with higher repetitions. Higher repetitions with lower resistance may be preferable for weaker, older, or higher-risk patients.

Number of Sets

The number of sets performed each session will depend upon the muscular fitness level of the participant, the rest intervals between stations, and the time allotted for the training session. The AACVPR (28) recommends that low-risk cardiac patients perform one to three sets of upper- and lower-body exercises per session, although the time allotment may not be sufficient for this amount of work and many patients may be limited by fatigue. Longer sessions have been associated with higher dropout rates, smaller additional gains in strength, increased hemodynamic parameters, increased fatigability, and an increased risk of musculoskeletal injuries (44, 80, 100, 103). Thus, it is best for your patients to perform one to two sets with proper form and increase the number of muscle groups they exercise, rather than to use fewer muscle groups and perform three sets of each exercise. Patients should not engage in multi-repetition sets to fatigue. The ACSM recommends that older subjects (i.e., > 60 years) perform only one set of upper/lower-body exercises (31). One set of multistation resistive exercise has been recommended since this lower volume of work has been shown to increase muscle thickness as effectively as three sets of resistive exercises in healthy subjects (104). Performance of one set of exercises for specified muscle groups with no time limit may be appropriate for strength gains in older patients, higher-risk patients, those with a low functional capacity, those who have time limitations, or those who fatigue easily.

Rate of Progression

As training occurs, you should have the patient achieve overload by first increasing the number of repetitions performed. Your patient should progress, over time, to no more than 15 repetitions per exercise. For some patients with more severe pathologies or lower functional capacities, you may wish to start with a higher number of repetitions and a lower level of resistance (e.g., 15 repetitions with resistance equivalent to 2.5 kg [5 lb]). When the patient can handle 12-15 repetitions at a given resistance comfortably at an RPE of 11-13, the weight may be increased to 5 kg (10 lb) (28). Once the individual can perform one to two sets at a desired resistance, you can also initiate progression by having the patient perform a third and final set (if time allows), or by again increasing the resistance. However, two sets should probably be the maximal volume for most patients. If elastic bands are used, the patient may progress by advancing to thicker bands with stronger tension over time. If hand weights or dumbbells are used, you can have the patient progress through a series of heavier weights over time.

Once the patient has performed a follow-up symptom-limited graded exercise test, he/she may be able to progress to an exercise equivalent of 60-80% of 1 RM if they are medically stable and have no orthopedic limitations (28, 41, 80). Patients who have been out of the program for a period of time should resume resistive training at no more than 50% of the intensity at which they had previously been training. Resistance should then be progressed in the same format as when the patient entered the program.

Determining Resistive-Training Workload

Many variations of resistive testing have been used in training protocols for estimating training workloads and exercise prescription in cardiac populations (8, 32, 41, 42, 45, 80). The 1 RM method has been most widely cited in cardiac research protocols. How safe is 1 RM testing for CRP participants? Studies that have monitored physiologic parameters (i.e., BP, HR, ECG) in properly screened patients have shown no significant ST-segment depression, serious arrhythmias, abnormal HR/BP responses, or sternotomy complications during resistive testing up to 100% of maximum voluntary contraction (19, 39-44, 55). In many of these studies, resistive testing was performed relatively early after the cardiac event. However, although 1 RM testing is apparently physiologically safe, its orthopedic safety has been questioned in older populations. Pollock et al. (103) concluded that 1 RM testing is probably inappropriate for older men and women who have joint problems specific to the muscle group being tested. Conversely, Shaw et al. (105) concluded that with proper preparation, 1 RM testing can be a safe assessment tool for the geriatric population. Gordon et al. (106) found 1 RM testing to be orthopedically and hemodynamically safe in younger, apparently healthy men and women aged 20-69 years. Wilke et al. (19) observed shoulder injuries in two cardiac patients during 1 RM upper-body testing performed at 4- and 12-week follow-up testing intervals, but both of these patients had a prior history of shoulder injuries. Research is needed in other clinical groups before maximal strength testing or 1 RM testing can be recommended for all CRP participants.

Since 1 RM or maximal voluntary contraction testing has been the standard form of assessment for determining training resistive workloads in many research studies, this type of testing may be suitable for many patients. However, most CRPs have a large percentage of older patients, and 1 RM testing may be inappropriate for certain individuals. If the 1 RM method (or a variation thereof) is selected for testing, use caution and screen participants carefully. Participants in CRPs should be warned against breath-holding during 1 RM testing and should not undergo testing if they have had recent orthopedic limitations or are at risk of musculoskeletal injury.

The ACSM (31) and others (33, 80, 100) have recommended an acclimation or "titration" technique for cardiac patients, which starts with the lightest weight or resistance on each resistive device. Patient responses are monitored for 10-12 repetitions to an RPE of 13-14 or "somewhat hard" on the Borg category scale. If the patient is asymptomatic and tolerates that workload well, the resistance is increased to a higher workload every 1-2 weeks. This technique facilitates better patient orientation, puts less initial stress on the patient, and may allow for a more accurate resistive exercise prescription. Staff may also prescribe training workloads by using the Borg category or category-ratio RPE scales alone. An RPE rating of 11-14 on the category scale or a 3-4 on the category-ratio scale during testing indicates a suitable initial training workload.

The 1 RM and titration methods just described are two of the more commonly used methods for determining resistive-training workloads in CRPs. There are other standard methods for assessing training workloads that may be more applicable to the individual patient (31, 38-47). It is ultimately up to the CRP staff to determine which resistive testing protocol is most suited for the person being tested.

Circuit Weight Training

A circuit training approach for resistive exercise has been widely recommended for cardiac patients because this type of exercise has been reported to be safer than free weights, easier to learn and participate in, and perhaps capable of eliciting significant gains in muscular strength and lean body weight (8, 29, 30, 32, 45). Circuit weight training may also enhance bone mineral content (especially in women), range of motion, cardiovascular endurance, and may provide additional benefits for the CRP participant through risk factor reduction (8, 9, 14, 29, 55, 107, 108). One of the benefits of using machines in a circuit fashion is the ability to start with low resistance and then progressively add small, incremental loads. The overload principle must be applied gradually for the safety and effectiveness of resistance training in cardiac populations. If your CRP cannot afford machines or has space limitations, you can develop excellent low-cost resistive circuits using a combination of dumbbells, elastics, barbells, free weights, wall pulleys, aerobic equipment, and even weighted "fanny" packs, plastic containers, or cloth bags. Each CWT program should be individualized and patients should move through the circuit at a moderate pace. Participants may also choose to simply perform machine or free-weight exercises over a longer time period, without emphasis on CWT. The parameters of CWT are presented in table 2.3.

Participants should perform circuit weight training on alternating days, 2-3 days per week, in conjunction with the regularly scheduled CRP sessions or under CRP staff supervision. Initially the patient should perform one circuit composed of 5–18 stations with low to moderate weight loads. Training workloads should be 30-60% of

Table 2.3   Circuit Weight Training Parameters for Cardiac Patients

CWT parameter	Cardiac recommendations
Resistance	**30-60% of 1 RM or low to moderate weight loads**
Repetitions	**8-20** 10-15 most often recommended
Exercise duration	**20-30 minutes**
Number of stations	**5-18**
Number of circuits/sets	**1-3** Depends upon patient's fitness level and time allotment for resistive exercise
Rest interval between stations	**≥ 30 seconds** Potential for greater improvement in cardiovascular endurance with shorter rest intervals Greater HR/BP recovery with longer rest intervals and less risk of cardiovascular complications
Speed of muscle contraction	**Lift to a count of 2, lower to a count of 4** Complete limb flexion/extension
Placement of CWT session	**After the CRP aerobic phase** Assures adequate warm-up, less risk of musculoskeletal injury, and prioritizes aerobic phase
Frequency Progression	**Alternating 2-3 days/week** **Increase resistance once 10-15 reps can be performed comfortably (RPE 11-13)** Increase sets depending upon time allotment for session, fitness level, and fatigability of the participant
Specificity	**All major muscle groups**

Reprinted with permission from D.E. Verrill and P.M. Ribisl, 1996, "Resistive exercise training in cardiac rehabilitation—an update," *Sports Medicine* 21(5):371.

1 RM if this method is being used to determine training resistance. Selected low-risk participants who are aerobically trained and medically stable may eventually progress to workloads corresponding to 60-80% of 1 RM (28).

Typically, patients should perform 8-15 repetitions per station with 30-60 second rest intervals between stations. Rest intervals of 30 seconds have been shown to facilitate higher $\dot{V}O_2$ levels than rest intervals of 60 seconds in healthy subjects (109). Rest periods of 60 seconds or more may allow for recovery of HR and BP between stations, but may also decrease the ability of the circuit to improve cardiovascular endurance. Since safety is of vital importance in CRPs, longer rest intervals or higher repetitions with lighter weights may be warranted for some patients. Each CWT session should last 20-30 minutes and should preferably be performed after the aerobic phase of the exercise session. There is little or no research on the risks or benefits of combining resistive and aerobic exercise intermittently during sessions, and this issue needs further study. Performing CWT after aerobic exercise assures adequate warm-up, less risk of muscular or orthopedic injury, and prioritization of the aerobic phase of the exercise session. During CWT sessions, patients should always exhale during the weight-lifting (concentric) phase of muscle contraction and inhale during the weight-lowering (eccentric) phase of muscle contraction. If your patients are confused by these instructions, tell them, "Breathe regularly while you lift" or "Count the repetitions out loud" to avoid the Valsalva maneuver.

To enhance joint mobility and reduce the risk of musculoskeletal injury, stretching and flexibility exercises should be performed before and/or after CWT sessions. All resistive training should be viewed as supplemental and should not be substituted for the aerobic phase of the exercise session. A summary of resistive-training instructions that may be distributed to patients is presented on page 76.

Regardless of the type of resistive-training equipment used, the circuit should include strengthening exercises for all major muscle groups (agonist-antagonist) and should be multijoint instead of single joint in nature. Your patients should exercise large muscle groups before small muscle groups and should alternate between upper- and lower-body exercises during resistive sessions. The exercises that are described on pages 68–73 should be included in the circuit.

Hemodynamic Monitoring

Heart rate and ventilatory responses in cardiac patients during resistive exercise depend on several factors, including

- the mode of resistive exercise,
- the amount of resistance,
- the volume of work (i.e., number of sets, stations, repetitions),
- the joint angle of contraction,
- the duration of rest intervals between exercises,
- the degree of Valsalva and/or isometric component,
- the cardiac impairment of the participant,
- the timing of actual measurements,
- body position, and
- prescribed medications (35, 36, 37, 39, 106, 109-111).

1. The rhomboids, teres, latissimus dorsi, posterior deltoids, and elbow flexors using movements similar to those for rowing.

2. The deltoid, triceps, and trapezius muscle groups using overhead press movements.

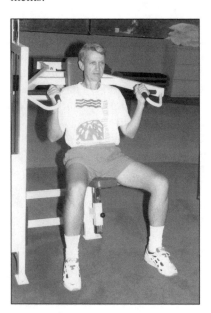 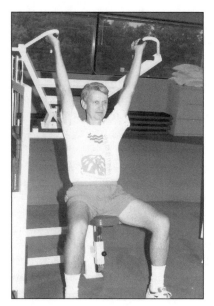

3. The pectoralis, latissimus dorsi, and elbow flexor muscles using pull-down movements.

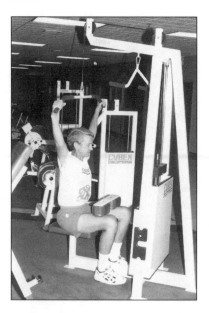 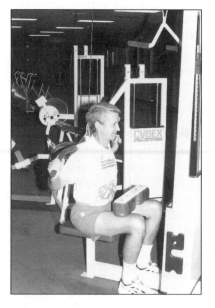

4.   The quadriceps muscles using knee flexion/extension.

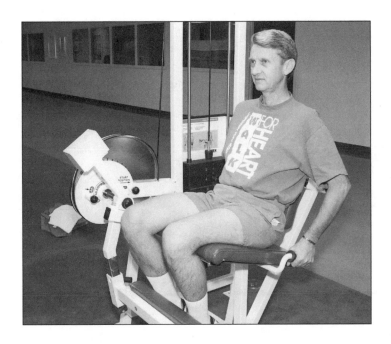

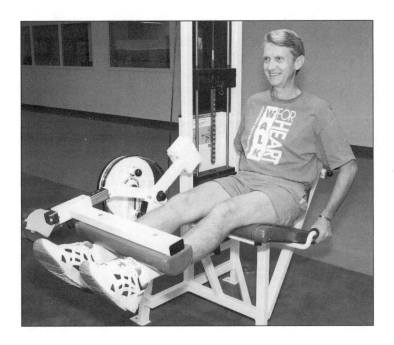

5.   The gluteus medius, anterior tibialis, and tensor fasciae latae muscles using lateral leg-raise exercises.

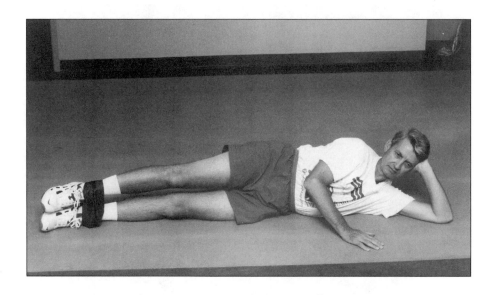

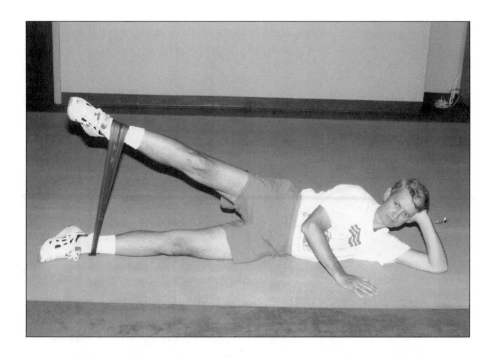

6. The gluteal and hamstring muscle groups using leg curl and/or leg press exercises.

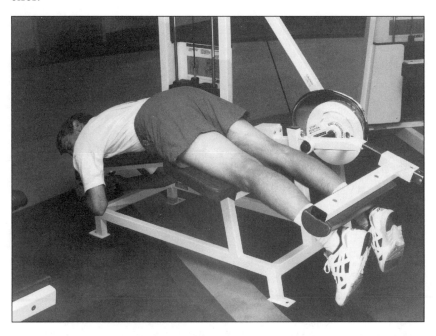

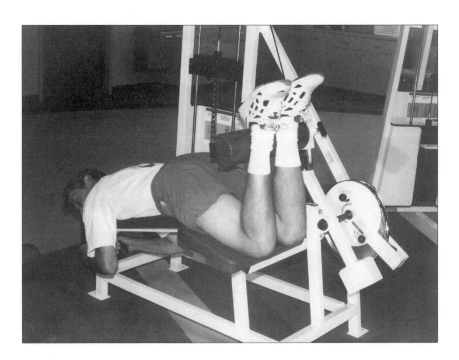

7.   The biceps muscles using biceps curl exercises.

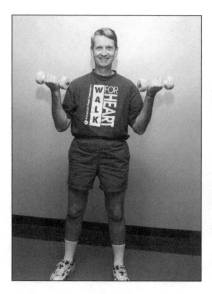 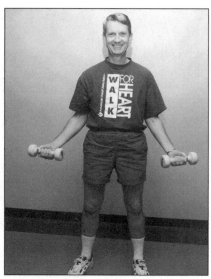

8.   The pectoral and triceps muscles with movements similar to those for push-ups and bench presses.

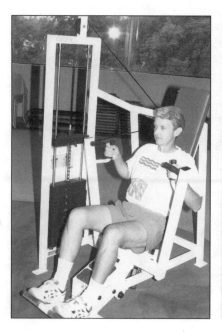 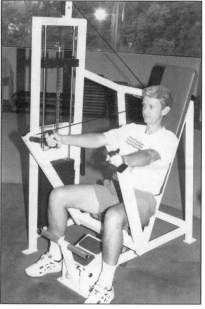

9. The posterior deltoid and triceps muscles using posterior arm-raise and shoulder "shrug" exercises.

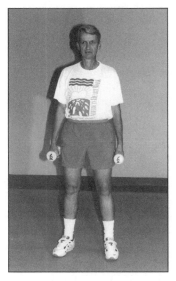 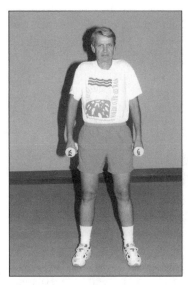

10. The abdominal and hip flexor muscles using pelvic tilt exercises, "crunches," abdominal resistance machines, or floor curl-up exercises.

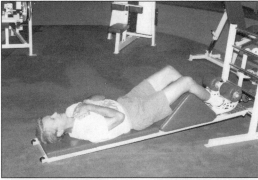

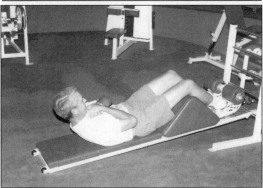

Generally, HR responses are significantly lower during resistive training than during aerobic training. Clinically acceptable elevations in systolic BP with somewhat higher diastolic BP responses have been reported during CWT protocols (8-16 repetitions at 30-60% of measured and predicted 1 RM) in selected cardiac patients (39, 42-45). But since both systolic and diastolic BP show a rapid decline after a weight lift (24, 34, 36, 37), some degree of hemodynamic monitoring during resistive training may be warranted for selected higher-risk patients to help identify cardiac insufficiency or arrhythmias.

The AACVPR (28) recommends BP and ECG monitoring for selected patients during resistive training, with more extensive monitoring in higher-risk individuals. The degree of hemodynamic monitoring will vary based upon the patient's risk stratification, cardiac pathology, and level of cardiovascular endurance. Too much monitoring could distract the patient from achieving the full benefits of resistive training and could promote more dependency on CRP staff. This would hinder attainment of improved self-efficacy and self-image.

The RPP has been shown to be a good indicator of myocardial oxygen consumption. Recording of HR and BP during muscle contraction may be valuable in some patients to provide an estimate of myocardial oxygen demand during resistive exercise (if measured). Blood pressure and HR measurements should be recorded during actual lifting movements for accurate hemodynamic assessment and RPP estimation. Because of the rapid drop in BP seen immediately after lifting, recordings taken at non–moving body sites (e.g., ankles) during lifting may provide an accurate measurement of arterial pressure. Because of limb movement, blood pressure often cannot be assessed accurately at the brachial artery during repetitive upper-body weight lifting. Thus, measurements can be taken in one arm while the patient continues to exercise with the other arm or with the legs. Blood pressure measurements may also be taken at the dorsalis pedis artery with a pneumatic cuff and Doppler stethoscope, and may provide greater accuracy and a better indication of arterial BP during upper-body resistive activities in patients predisposed to hypertensive or hypotensive episodes (17, 44). Staff may need to monitor some patients for postural hypotensive changes as they move from station to station.

Intensity violators of prescribed target HRs or people with complex dysrhythmias may benefit from periodic "quick-check" rhythm strip checks, radiotelemetry, or ambulatory Holter monitoring. In general, when performing resistive exercise, patients should not elicit HR responses greater than those observed at 85% of $\dot{V}O_2max$ or at the ischemic threshold from the symptom-limited graded exercise test (44). Those who are at higher risk of cardiac complications or who cannot monitor their HR because of physical or intellectual impairment may also benefit from ECG monitoring to assure accurate HR estimation and arrhythmia documentation (112). Since the RPP can be calculated accurately if HR and BP are recorded during actual lifting movements, this measure may provide a better indication of cardiovascular stress than either HR or BP alone. Resistive training will elicit an increase in RPP through a higher systolic pressure response, while HR may be lower than with traditional aerobic exercise. The resistive activity recording form should include, within the patient's resistive exercise prescription, the RPP at which signs or symptoms of myocardial ischemia or cardiac insufficiency appear during symptom-limited graded exercise.

Until further research has been published, it may be best to take a prudent approach and monitor high-risk patients more vigilantly, especially during the early resistive-training sessions. However, no additional monitoring or staff supervision is necessary for resistive exercise than is required for a normal CRP session. Less hemodynamic monitoring will probably become the norm for most patients. Presently, low-risk or stable patients require no additional cardiovascular monitoring during resistive exercise.

Patient Instruction and Safety

Proper instruction is important to assure that the CRP participant performs resistive exercise in a safe and mechanically efficient manner and with a low risk of musculoskeletal injury or adverse cardiac events. Distribute the "Resistive Exercise Instructions for Cardiac Participants" (page 76) to each patient, or post a copy (preferably enlarged) in a prominent place in your workout facility. The following are suggestions summarized from published guidelines on cardiac weight training for optimal patient instruction and safety during resistive training (28-33).

1. Make sure that an exercise specialist, physical therapist, or athletic trainer thoroughly orients CRP participants to each modality or piece of equipment. Perform the initial orientation and testing on an individual basis to assure that each patient learns to perform the exercises safely and efficiently. Allow ample time for questions, testing, and practice on each modality during the initial exercise session. Provide a complete description of the mechanical function of each piece of apparatus and show the correct body position. Also provide clear warnings about the risk of improper usage.

2. Instruct patients to maintain a loose, comfortable grip during muscle contraction on each piece of equipment or to perform the lift with the palm/fingers extended to reduce pure isometric components. Tell them to avoid sustained hand gripping on other pieces of resistive equipment (e.g., bands, dumbbells). Rather than gripping elastic bands, they should wrap the bands around their hands for tension. In the initial training sessions, emphasize proper breathing technique (i.e., exhalation with exertion) and the dangers of the Valsalva maneuver.

3. Have the patients perform each exercise through a full range of motion (or in their "pain-free" zone) with each resistive modality. Range-of-motion limitation may be warranted for some patients with orthopedic limitations. Machine weights, if used, should be raised with slow, controlled movements to a count of two and lowered gradually to a count of four. Large muscle groups should be exercised before small muscle groups for both the upper and lower body. Tell the patient that he/she is responsible for log recording of weight lifted, repetitions, and any physiological measurements taken on individual machines or with resistive modalities.

4. Participants should perform stretching/flexibility exercises before and/or after CWT sessions to enhance joint mobility and reduce the risk of injury. Increase muscle temperature through warm-up to allow for optimal joint range of motion. Flexibility may be enhanced with some resistive devices.

Resistive Exercise Instructions
for Cardiac Participants[1]

1. Participate in the aerobic exercise session or perform at least a 10-minute full-body warm-up before each resistive exercise session.

2. Breathe normally or exhale during muscle contraction. Do not hold your breath.

3. Maintain a loose, comfortable grip during muscle contraction on each piece of equipment.

4. Perform lifting movements through a complete range of motion.

5. Lift the weight smoothly to a count of two and lower slowly to a count of four.

6. Exercise all major muscle groups and work large muscles before small muscles.

7. Learn and practice proper technique and form for each piece of apparatus. Ask questions to be sure you understand proper usage of equipment at each station.

8. Never drop the dumbbells, hand weights, or machine weights.

9. Avoid injury by adhering to the instructions of the cardiac rehabilitation staff.

10. Terminate resistive exercise if you develop symptoms of intolerance such as chest pain, dizziness, faintness, or fatigue.

11. Record your rating of perceived exertion (6-20 RPE scale) on each piece of equipment. You should perceive the resistive effort as light (11) to somewhat hard (14) during exertion at each station.

12. Record the amount of resistance (e.g., color of elastic band, number of plates on the machine) at each station. Also record the number of repetitions you perform on each piece of apparatus.

[1]Reprinted with permission from D.E. Verrill and P.M. Ribisl, 1996, "Resistive exercise training in cardiac rehabilitation—an update," *Sports Medicine* 21(5):353.

Criteria for Termination of a
Resistive Exercise Session[1]

1. Acute MI or suspicion of MI

2. Signs of poor perfusion including pallor, cyanosis, or cold and clammy skin

3. Central nervous symptoms including ataxia, vertigo, visual or gait problems

4. Light-headedness, confusion, nausea, or severe peripheral circulating insufficiency

5. Onset of angina with resistive exercise

6. Drop in systolic BP accompanied by signs/symptoms or drop below standing resting pressure

7. Excessive BP rise measured during lifting: systolic $\geq$ 220 mmHg or diastolic $\geq$ 110 mmHg

8. Inappropriate bradycardia (decrease in HR > 10 beats $\cdot$ min^{-1}) during resistive exercise

9. Supraventricular tachycardia or exercise-induced complex supraventricular dysrhythmias

10. Pronounced ST segment changes ($\geq$ 2-3 mm) from rest on the basis of telemetered ECG recordings

11. Onset of frequent ventricular ectopy and/or ventricular tachycardia (three or more consecutive PVCs)

12. Exercise-induced left bundle branch block that cannot be distinguished from a wide QRS tachycardia

13. Severe dyspnea, wheezing, or fatigue

14. Onset of second- and/or third-degree atrioventricular block from telemetry or "quick-look" recordings

15. New onset or aggravation of a preexisting musculoskeletal problem that would prohibit continuation of the resistive session

16. Failure to comply with exercise prescription, proper lifting technique, and/or appropriate log recording (i.e., recording of physiological parameters, amount of resistance, number of repetitions)

17. Discomfort related to past surgery (e.g., CABG, rotator cuff)

18. Rating of 18 or above on the Borg category RPE scale

[1]Reprinted with permission from D.E. Verrill and P.M. Ribisl, 1996, "Resistive exercise training in cardiac rehabilitation—an update," *Sports Medicine* 21(5):375.

5. Terminate resistive exercise for the same reasons you would terminate aerobic exercise. A summary of termination criteria adapted from the AACVPR (28), ACSM/ACP (31), and AHA (92) standards is presented on page 77. Strict observation for common cardiac symptoms, such as angina, dizziness, syncope, palpitations, and fatigue, should be followed. An excessive rise or drop in BP or the development of significant dysrhythmias warrants termination of the resistive exercise session. Although cardiovascular complications are rare with this mode of training, patients must learn to monitor their own symptoms and to report any unusual symptomatology to the CRP staff. Be sure to encourage patients to become self-sufficient in this respect, and see that they do not rely strictly on CRP staff for continuous monitoring or supervision during resistive training.

6. Have a fully equipped crash cart, defibrillator, oxygen, and all necessary emergency equipment readily available in the event of cardiopulmonary complications. Advanced cardiac life support-trained personnel should be ready to respond to emergency situations. Perform periodic drills with simulated code situations in the resistive-training area on a regular rotating basis.

7. During the early resistive exercise sessions, do not have the patient exceed an RPE of 15 on the Borg category scale or a 5 on the category-ratio scale. Generally, RPE values should range from "fairly light" (11) to "somewhat hard" (14) on the category scale or from "moderate" (2) to "difficult" (4) on the category-ratio scale. As the patient adapts to resistive exercise, the RPE values may progress to "hard" (15-16) on the category scale or "difficult to more difficult" (5-7) on the category-ratio scale (113). Have the patient record his/her RPE each session for modification of weight progression.

8. Designate a staff person (i.e., exercise specialist, athletic trainer, physical therapist) to supervise the resistive-training area during cardiac resistive exercise. He/she should ensure that the patient is using proper training technique and is following the exercise prescription. This staff person should also ensure that HR and BP, if taken, are being measured accurately during muscle contraction.

9. Be aware of any musculoskeletal limitations (e.g., bursitis, tendinitis) that may be present, and modify the patient's training regimen to accommodate limitations. Never let your patients participate in resistive exercise during periods of acute pain or inflammation.

10. Periodically review the patient's exercise logs to monitor rate of progression, and specify changes in the resistive exercise regimen. Resistive progression will vary depending upon the patient's functional capacity, cardiovascular status, body weight, and strength. Generally, advancement of resistance should be no greater than 2.2 kg (5 lb) for arm exercise and up to 4.5 kg (10 lb) for leg exercise per session.

11. Maintain the resistive equipment on a regular schedule of preventive maintenance, and clean the equipment frequently. Adhere to established guidelines for care and maintenance for all equipment, and prioritize risk management for patient safety. Before beginning the program, participants in CRPs should have knowledge of any potential risks of using resistive equipment (114-115).

Conclusions

Cardiopulmonary rehabilitation programs are designed to enhance the quality of life and modify CAD risk factors so that participants may return to everyday job duties and recreational pursuits as soon as possible after a cardiac event. The major goal of resistive training is for the patient to develop sufficient muscular fitness to return to a physically independent lifestyle. Restoration of muscular strength and range of motion to resume daily living habits is essential for all patients, particularly the elderly. Since most daily activities involve upper- and lower-body movements, resistive exercise training should play a very significant role in all CRPs. Appropriately prescribed resistive exercise has been shown to be safe for cardiac patients, even at relatively high workloads. Resistive exercise has not been shown to exacerbate HR or systolic BP responses beyond clinically acceptable levels in cardiac patients. However, diastolic BP may be greater than that observed during aerobic exercise. The benefits or risks of higher diastolic BPs during resistive exercise remain to be seen.

Circuit weight training has been shown to improve strength, bone mass, lean body mass, and self-efficacy and to decrease some risk factors for CAD. Many studies have provided evidence that CWT, when combined with aerobic exercise, provides beneficial central and/or peripheral cardiovascular adaptations over those seen with aerobic training alone. However, CWT may not supply the needed stimulus to beneficially alter BP or lipid/lipoprotein levels. Since few investigators have examined long-term resistive-training adaptations in cardiac or high-risk populations, further research is needed to examine the effects of chronic resistive exercise on blood chemistry and other CAD risk factors.

Overall, there are numerous benefits with little risk of untoward events for participants of properly supervised cardiac resistive training programs. Whereas many recent studies have focused on cardiac populations, questions remain regarding cardiac resistive exercise. Some of these questions are:

- Should high-risk patients perform CWT?
- Can patients safely perform resistive training intermittently with aerobic training?
- How safe is 1 RM testing for older cardiac patients or special cardiac populations?
- What are the acute and long-term cardiovascular and metabolic effects of resistive exercise in patients with impaired LV function, cardiac/lung transplant, cancer, renal disease, obstructive lung disease, and diabetes?
- Should resistive-training principles and modalities differ for female cardiac patients?
- What types of guidelines should be required for those who wish to perform continuous isodynamic exercise?

Future investigators should continue to incorporate continuous invasive and noninvasive cardiovascular monitoring techniques to fully assess the risks, benefits, and complication rates of resistive exercise in higher-risk subjects and to provide recommendations for these patients. At present, CRP personnel may safely prescribe resistive exercise for most of their participants. This kind of risk factor intervention will encourage lifetime behavior changes, improve strength and endurance, improve self-image, and better prepare the patient to return to daily strength tasks safely, more efficiently, and with greater self-confidence.

References

1. Painter, P., and Hanson, P. Isometric exercise: implications for the cardiac patient. In L.K. Hall and G.C. Meyer (Eds.), *Cardiac rehabilitation: exercise testing and prescription* (pp. 223-242). Champaign, IL: Life Enhancement; 1984.

2. Ferguson, R.J., Cote, P., Bourassa, M.G., and Corbara, F. Coronary blood flow during isometric and dynamic exercise in angina pectoris patients. *Journal of Cardiac Rehabilitation,* **1**, 21-27; 1981.

3. Wenger, N.K., and Hellerstein, H.K. *Rehabilitation of the coronary patient.* New York: Churchill Livingston; 1992.

4. Hurley, B.F. Strength training in the elderly to enhance health status. *Medicine, Exercise, Nutrition, and Health,* **4**, 217-229; 1995.

5. Haennel, R.G., Quinney, H.A., and Kappagoda, C.T. Effects of hydraulic circuit training following coronary artery bypass surgery. *Medicine and Science in Sports and Exercise,* **23**, 158-165; 1991.

6. Hurley, B.F., and Kokkinos, P.F. Effects of weight training on risk factors for coronary artery disease. *Sports Medicine,* **4**, 231-238; 1987.

7. Hurley, B.F., Hagberg, J.M., Goldberg, A.P., Seals, D.R., Ehsani, A.A., Brennan, R.E., and Holloszy, J.O. Resistive training can reduce coronary risk factors without altering $\dot{V}O_2$max or percent body fat. *Medicine and Science in Sports and Exercise,* **20**, 150-154; 1988.

8. Kelemen, M.H., Stewart, K.J., Gillilan, R.E., Ewart, C.K., Valenti, S.A., Manley, J.D., and Kelemen, M.D. Circuit weight training in cardiac patients. *Journal of the American College of Cardiology,* **7**, 38-42; 1986.

9. McCartney, N., McKelvie, R.S., Haslam, D.R.S., and Jones, N.L. Usefulness of weightlifting training in improving strength and maximal power output in coronary artery disease. *American Journal of Cardiology,* **67**, 939-945; 1991.

10. Smutok, M.A., Reece, C., Kokkinos, P.F., Farmer, C., Dawson, P., Shulman, R., DeVane-Bell, J., Patterson, J., Charabogos, C., Goldberg, A.P., and Hurley, B.F. Aerobic versus strength training for risk factor intervention in middle-aged men at high risk for coronary artery disease. *Metabolism,* **42**, 177-184; 1993.

11. Ewart, C.K., Stewart, K.J., Gillilan, R.E., and Kelemen, M.H. Self-efficacy mediates strength gains during circuit weight training in men with coronary artery disease. *Medicine and Science in Sports and Exercise,* **18**, 531-540; 1987.

12. Ewart, C.K. Psychological effects of resistive weight training: implications for cardiac patients. *Medicine and Science in Sports and Exercise,* **21**, 683-688; 1989.

13. Brown, A.B., McCartney, N., and Sale, D.G. Positive adaptations to weight-lifting training in the elderly. *Journal of Applied Physiology,* **69**, 1725-1733; 1990.

14. Hurley, B.F., Seals, D.R., Ehsani, A.A., Cartier, L.J., Dalsky, G.P., Hagberg, J.M., and Holloszy, J.O. Effects of high-intensity strength training on cardiovascular function. *Medicine and Science in Sports and Exercise,* **16**, 483-488; 1984.

15. Ballor, D.L., Katch, V.L., Becque, M.D., and Marks, C.R. Resistance weight training during caloric restriction enhances lean body weight maintenance. *American Journal of Clinical Nutrition,* **47**, 19-25; 1988.

16. Fletcher, G.F., Blair, S.N., Blumenthal, J., Caspersen, C., Chaitman, B., Epstein, S., Falls, H., Froelicher, E.S.S., Froelicher, V., and Pina, I.L. American Heart Association statement on exercise—benefits and recommendations for physical activity programs for all Americans. *Circulation,* **86**, 340-344; 1992.

17. Franklin, B.A., Bonzheim, K., Gordon, S., and Timmis, G.C. Resistance training in cardiac rehabilitation. *Journal of Cardiopulmonary Rehabilitation,* **11**, 99-107; 1991.

18. Hanson, P., and Nagle, F. Isometric exercise: cardiovascular responses in normal and cardiac populations. *Cardiology Clinics,* **5**, 157-170; 1987.

19. Wilke, N.A., Sheldahl, L.M., Levandoski, S.G., Hoffman, M.D., Dougherty, S.M., and Tristani, F.E. Transfer effect of upper extremity training to weight carrying in men with ischemic heart disease. *Journal of Cardiopulmonary Rehabilitation,* **11**, 365-372; 1991.

20. DeBusk, R., Valdez, R., and Houston, N. Cardiovascular response to dynamic and static effort soon after myocardial infarction: application to occupational work assessment. *Circulation,* **58**, 368-375; 1978.

21. Markiewicz, W., Houston, N., and DeBusk, R. A comparison of static and dynamic exercise soon after myocardial infarction. *Israeli Journal of Medical Science,* **15**, 894-897; 1979.

22. Rod, J.L., Braun, J.Q., Rehm, L.M., and Landes, J.R. Simulated work activity in patients with coronary artery disease: a clinical protocol. *Journal of Cardiopulmonary Rehabilitation,* **9**, 439-444; 1989.

23. Schram, V., and Hanson, P. Cardiovascular and metabolic responses to weight-loaded walking in cardiac rehabilitation patients. *Journal of Cardiopulmonary Rehabilitation,* **8**, 28-32; 1988.

24. Sheldahl, L.M., Wilke, N.A., Tristani, F.E., and Kalbfleisch, J.H. Response to repetitive static-dynamic exercise in patients with coronary artery disease. *Journal of Cardiac Rehabilitation,* **5**, 139-145; 1985.

25. Taylor, J.L., Copeland, R.B., Cousins, A.L., Kansal, S., Roitman, D., and Sheffield, L.T. The effect of isometric exercise on the graded exercise test in patients with stable angina pectoris. *Journal of Cardiac Rehabilitation,* **1**, 450-458; 1981.

26. Wilke, N.A., Sheldahl, L.M., Levandoski, S.G., Hoffman, M.D., and Tristani, F.E. Weight carrying versus handgrip exercise testing in men with coronary artery disease. *American Journal of Cardiology,* **64**, 736-740; 1989.

27. Sheldahl, L.M., Levandoski, S.G., Wilke, N.A., Dougherty, S.M., and Tristani, F.E. Responses of patients with coronary artery disease to common carpentry tasks. *Journal of Cardiopulmonary Rehabilitation,* **13**, 283-290; 1993.

28. American Association of Cardiovascular and Pulmonary Rehabilitation. *Guidelines for cardiac rehabilitation programs* (2nd ed.). Champaign, IL: Human Kinetics; 1995.

29. Gettman, L.R., and Pollock, M.L. Circuit weight training: a critical review of its physiological benefits. *Physician and Sportsmedicine,* **9**, 44-60; 1981.

30. Kelemen, M.H. Resistive training safety and assessment guidelines for cardiac and coronary prone patients. *Medicine and Science in Sports and Exercise,* **21**, 675-677; 1989.

31. American College of Sports Medicine. *Guidelines for exercise testing and prescription* (5th ed.). Philadelphia: Williams & Wilkins; 1995.

32. Sparling, P.B., and Cantwell, J.D. Strength training guidelines for cardiac patients. *Physician and Sportsmedicine,* **17**, 190-196; 1989.

33. Verrill, D., and Ribisl, P. Resistive exercise training in cardiac rehabilitation—an update. *Sports Medicine,* **21**, 347-383; 1996.

34. MacDougall, J.D., Tuxen, D., Sale, D.G., Moroz, J.R., and Sutton, J.R. Arterial blood pressure response to heavy resistance exercise. *Journal of Applied Physiology,* **58**, 785-790; 1985.

35. Mitchell, J.H., Schibye, B., Payne, F.C., and Saltin, B. Response of arterial blood pressure to static exercise in relation to muscle mass, force development, and electromyographic activity. *Circulation Research,* **48**(Suppl. 1):70-76; 1981.

36. Haslam, D.R.S., McCartney, N., McKelvie, R.S., and MacDougall, J.D. Direct measurement of arterial blood pressure during formal weightlifting in cardiac patients. *Journal of Cardiopulmonary Rehabilitation,* **8**, 213-225; 1988.

37. Wiecek, E.M., McCartney, N., McKelvie, R.S., and MacDougall, D. Comparison of direct and indirect measures of systemic arterial pressure during weightlifting in coronary artery disease. *American Journal of Cardiology,* **66**, 1065-1069; 1990.

38. Stewart, K.J., Mason, M., and Kelemen, M.H. Three-year participation in circuit weight training improves muscular strength and self-efficacy in cardiac patients. *Journal of Cardiopulmonary Rehabilitation,* **8**, 292-296; 1988.

39. Butler, R.M., Beierwaltes, W.H., and Rogers, F.J. The cardiovascular response to circuit weight training in patients with cardiac disease. *Journal of Cardiopulmonary Rehabilitation,* **7**, 402-409; 1987.

40. Featherstone, J.F., Holly, R.G., and Amsterdam, E.A. Physiologic responses to weight lifting in coronary artery disease. *American Journal of Cardiology,* **71**, 287-292; 1993.

41. Ghilarducci, L.E., Holly, R.G., and Amsterdam, E.A. Effects of high resistance training in coronary artery disease. *American Journal of Cardiology,* **64**, 866-870; 1989.

42. Sparling, P.B., Cantwell, J.D., Dolan, C.M., and Niederman, R.K. Strength training in a cardiac rehabilitation program: a six-month follow up. *Archives of Physical Medicine and Rehabilitation,* **71**, 148-152; 1990.

43. Squires, R.W., Muri, A.J., Anderson, L.J., Allison, T.G., Miller, T.D., and Gau, G.T. Weight training during Phase II (early outpatient) cardiac rehabilitation. *Journal of Cardiopulmonary Rehabilitation,* **11**, 360-364; 1991.

44. Stralow, C.R., Ball, T.E., and Looney, M. Acute cardiovascular responses of patients with coronary disease to dynamic variable resistance exercise of different intensities. *Journal of Cardiopulmonary Rehabilitation,* **13**, 255-263; 1993.

45. Vander, L.B., Franklin, B.A., Wrisley, D., and Rubenfire, M. Acute cardiovascular responses to Nautilus exercise in cardiac patients: implications for exercise training. *Annals of Sports Medicine,* **2**, 165-169; 1986.

46. Cononie, C.C., Graves, J.E., Pollock, M.L., Phillips, M.I., Sumners, C., and Hagberg, J.M. Effect of exercise training on blood pressure in 70- to 79-year old men and women. *Medicine and Science in Sports and Exercise,* **23**, 505-511; 1991.

47. Fiatarone, M.A., Marks, E.C., Ryan, N.D., Meredith, C.N., Lipsitz, L.A., and Evans, W.J. High intensity strength training in nonagenarians. *Journal of the American Medical Association,* **263**, 3029-3034; 1990.

48. Frontera, W.R., Meredith, C.N., O'Reilly, K.P., Knuttgen, H.G., and Evans, W.J. Strength conditioning in older men: skeletal muscle hypertrophy and improved function. *Journal of Applied Physiology,* **64**, 1038-1044; 1988.

49. Parsons, D., Sherrill, K., Foster, V., and Oliva, P. Strength training improves balance and endurance for seniors. *Your Patient and Fitness,* **7**, 21-24; 1993.

50. Goldberg, A.P. Aerobic and resistive exercise modify risk factors for coronary heart disease. *Medicine and Science in Sports and Exercise,* **21**, 669-674; 1989.

51. Svedahl, K., Haennel, R.G., Hudec, R., Habib, N., and Gebhart, V. The effects of circuit training on the physical fitness of post-myocardial infarction (MI) patients. *Medicine and Science in Sports and Exercise,* **26**(Suppl. 1):185; 1994 (abstract).

52. Blumenthal, J.A., Siegel, W.C., and Appelbaum, M. Failure of exercise to reduce blood pressure in patients with mild hypertension. *Journal of the American Medical Association,* **266**, 2098-2104; 1991.

53. Stewart, K.J., McFarland, L.D., Weinhofer, J.J., Brown, C., and Shapiro, E.P. Weight training soon after myocardial infarction. *Medicine and Science in Sports and Exercise,* **26**(Suppl. 1): 32; 1994 (abstract).

54. Butler, R.M., Palmer, G., and Rogers, F.J. Circuit weight training in early cardiac rehabilitation. *Journal of the American Osteopathic Association,* **1**, 77-89; 1992.

55. Daub, W.D., Knapik, G.P., and Black, W.R. Strength training early after myocardial infarction. *Journal of Cardiopulmonary Rehabilitation,* **16**, 100-108; 1996.

56. Kokkinos, P.F., Hurley, B.F., Smutok, M.A., Farmer, C., Reece, C., Shulman, R., Charabogos, C., Patterson, J., Will, S., Devane-Bell, J., and Goldberg, A.P. Strength training does not improve lipoprotein-lipid profiles in men at risk for CHD. *Medicine and Science in Sports and Exercise,* **23**, 1134-1139; 1991.

57. Wallace, M.B., Moffatt, R.J., Haymes, E.M., and Green, N.R. Acute effects of resistance exercise on parameters of lipoprotein metabolism. *Medicine and Science in Sports and Exercise,* **23**, 199-204; 1991.

58. Boyden, T.W., Pamenter, R.W., and Going, S.G. Resistance exercise training is associated with decreases in serum low-density lipoprotein cholesterol levels in premenopausal women. *Archives of Internal Medicine,* **153**, 97-100; 1993.

59. Lampman, R.M., and Schteingart, D.E. Effects of exercise training on glucose control, lipid metabolism, and insulin sensitivity in hypertriglyceridemia and non-insulin dependent diabetes mellitus. *Medicine and Science in Sports and Exercise,* **23**, 703-712; 1991.

60. Mikines, K.J., Sonne, B., and Farrell, P.A. Effect of physical exercise on sensitivity and responsiveness to insulin in humans. *American Journal of Physiology,* **254**, 248-259; 1988.

61. Saito, M., Yamazaki, T., Goto, Y., Sumiyoshi, T., Fukami, K., Haze, K., and Hiramori, K. Cardiovascular responses during ordinary activities in healthy subjects: predominance of blood pressure response over heart rate in activities with isometric components. *Journal of Cardiopulmonary Rehabilitation,* **7**, 253-258; 1987.

62. Fardy, P.S. Isometric exercise and the cardiovascular system. *Physician and Sportmedicine,* **9**, 42-56; 1981.
63. Lind, A.R., and McNicol, G.W. Circulatory responses to sustained handgrip contractions performed during other exercises, both rhythmic and static. *Journal of Physiology,* **192**, 595-607; 1976.
64. Misner, J.E., Going, S.B., Massey, B.H., Ball, T.E., Bemben, M.G., and Hall, M.D. Cardiovascular response to sustained maximal voluntary static muscle contraction. *Medicine and Science in Sports and Exercise,* **22**, 194-199; 1990.
65. Lewis, S.F., Snell, P.G., and Taylor, W.F. Role of muscle mass and mode of contraction in circulatory responses to exercise. *Journal of Applied Physiology,* **58**, 146-151; 1985.
66. Atkins, J.M., Matthews, O.A., Blomqvist, C.G., and Mullins, C.B. Incidence of arrhythmias induced by isometric and dynamic exercise. *British Heart Journal,* **38**, 465-471; 1976.
67. Elkayam, U., Roth, A., Weber, L., Hsueh, W., and Naima, M. Isometric exercise in patients with chronic advanced heart failure: hemodynamic and neurohumoral evaluation. *Circulation,* **72**, 975-981; 1985.
68. Keren, G., Katz, S., Gage, J., Strom, J., and Sonnenblick, E.H. Effect of isometric exercise on cardiac performance and mitral regurgitation in patients with severe congestive heart failure. *American Heart Journal,* **118**, 973-979; 1989.
69. Kerber, R.E., Miller, R.A., and Najjar, S.M. Myocardial ischemic effects of isometric, dynamic and combined exercise in coronary artery disease. *Chest,* **67**, 388-394; 1975.
70. Sagiv, M., Hanson, P., Besozzi, M., Nagle, F., and Zager, L. Left ventricular responses to upright isometric handgrip and deadlift in men with coronary artery disease. *American Journal of Cardiology,* **55**, 1298-1302; 1985.
71. Lowe, D.K., Rothbaum, D.A., McHenry, P.L., Corya, B.C., and Knoebel, S.B. Myocardial blood flow response to isometric (handgrip) and treadmill exercise in coronary artery disease. *Circulation,* **51**, 126-131; 1975.
72. DeBusk, R., Pitts, W., Haskell, W., and Houston, N. Comparison of cardiovascular responses to static-dynamic efforts and dynamic effort alone in patients with chronic ischemic heart disease. *Circulation,* **59**, 977-984; 1979.
73. Haissly, J.C., Messin, R., Degre, S., Vandermoten, P., Demaret, B., and Simpson, H. Comparative response to isometric (static) and dynamic exercise tests in coronary disease. *American Journal of Cardiology,* **33**, 791-796; 1974.
74. Landi, J., Wygand, J., Otto, R., Kramer, J., Helgemoe, S., Calarco, L., and Bideaux, A. Hemodynamic and metabolic responses to two modes of load transport in patients with cardiac disease. *Journal of Cardiopulmonary Rehabilitation,* **14**, 43-46; 1994.
75. Sheldahl, L.M., Wilke, N.A., Tristani, F.E., and Kalbfleisch, J.H. Response of patients after myocardial infarction to carrying a graded series of weight loads. *American Journal of Cardiology,* **52**, 698-703; 1983.
76. MacGowan, G.A., Murali, S., Loftus, S., and Posner, J.D. Comparison of metabolic, ventilatory, and neurohumoral responses during light forearm isometric exercise and isotonic exercise in congestive heart failure. *American Journal of Cardiology,* **77**, 390-396; 1996.

77. Dougherty, S.M., Sheldahl, L.M., Wilke, N.A., Levandoski, S.G., Hoffman, M.D., and Tristani, F.E. Physiologic responses to shoveling and thermal stress in men with cardiac disease. *Medicine and Science in Sports and Exercise*, **25**, 790-795; 1993.

78. Sheldahl, L.M., Wilke, N.A., Dougherty, S.M., Levandoski, S.G., Hoffman, M.D., and Tristani, F.E. Effect of age and coronary artery disease on response to snow shoveling. *Journal of the American College of Cardiology*, **20**, 1111-1117; 1992.

79. Franklin, B.A., Hogan, P., Bonzheim, K., Bakalyar, D., Terrien, E., Gordon, S., and Timmis, G.C. Cardiac demands of heavy snow shoveling. *Journal of the American Medical Association*, **273**, 880-882; 1995.

80. Pollock, M.L., Welsch, M.A., and Graves, J.E. Exercise prescription for cardiac rehabilitation. In M.L. Pollock and D.H. Schmidt (Eds.), *Heart disease and rehabilitation* (pp. 265-266). Champaign, IL: Human Kinetics; 1995.

81. Walter, P.R., Porcari, J.P., Brice, G., and Terry, L. Acute responses to using walking poles in patients with coronary artery disease. *Journal of Cardiopulmonary Rehabilitation*, **16**, 245-250; 1996.

82. Graves, J.E., Martin, A.D., Miltenberger, L.A., and Pollock, M.L. Physiological responses to walking with hand weights, wrist weights, and ankle weights. *Medicine and Science in Sports and Exercise*, **20**, 265-271; 1988.

83. Graves, J.E., Pollock, M.L., Montain, S.J., Jackson, A.S., and O'Keefe, J.M. The effect of hand-held weights on the physiological responses to walking exercise. *Medicine and Science in Sports and Exercise*, **19**, 260-265; 1987.

84. Graves, J.E., Sagiv, M., Pollock, M.L., and Miltenberger, L.A. Effect of hand-held weights and wrist weights on the metabolic and hemodynamic responses to submaximal exercise in hypertensive responders. *Journal of Cardiopulmonary Rehabilitation*, **8**, 134-140; 1988.

85. Evans, B.W., Potteiger, J.A., Bray, M.C., and Tuttle, J.L. Metabolic and hemodynamic responses to walking with hand weights in older individuals. *Medicine and Science in Sports and Exercise*, **26**, 1047-1052; 1994.

86. Amos, K.R., Porcari, J.P., Bauer, S.R., and Wilson, P.K. The safety and effectiveness of walking with ankle weights and wrist weights for patients with cardiovascular disease. *Journal of Cardiopulmonary Rehabilitation*, **12**, 254-260; 1992.

87. Auble, T.E., Schwartz, L., and Robertson, R.J. Aerobic requirements for moving handweights through various ranges of motion while walking. *Physician and Sportsmedicine*, **15**, 133-140; 1987.

88. Garber, C.E., Fiske, C.H., Manfredi, T.G., and Heller, G.V. Circulatory responses to walking and jogging exercise with hand-held weights in young women. *Medicine, Exercise, Nutrition, and Health*, **1**, 92-96; 1992.

89. Maud, P.J., Stokes, G.D., and Stokes, L.R. Stride frequency, perceived exertion, and oxygen cost response to walking with variations in arm swing and hand held weight. *Journal of Cardiopulmonary Rehabilitation*, **10**, 294-299; 1990.

90. Miller, J.F., and Stamford, B.A. Intensity and energy cost of weighted walking vs. running for men and women. *Journal of Applied Physiology*, **62**, 1497-1501; 1987.

91. Zarandona, J.E., Nelson, A.G., Conlee, R.K., and Fisher, A.G. Physiological responses to hand-carried weights. *Physician and Sportsmedicine*, **14**, 113-120; 1986.

92. Fletcher, G.F., Balady, G., Froelicher, V.F., Hartley, L.H., Haskell, W.L., and Pollock, M.L. Exercise standards—a statement for healthcare professionals from the American Heart Association. *Circulation*, **91**, 580-615; 1995.

93. Campbell, B.F., Sheldahl, L., Wilke, N., Dougherty, S., Levandoski, S., and Tristani, F. Effects of upper extremity blood distribution on weight carrying in men with ischemic heart disease. *Journal of Cardiopulmonary Rehabilitation*, **13**, 37-42; 1993.

94. Wilke, N.A., Sheldahl, L.M., Tristani, F.E., and Hughes, C.V. The safety of static-dynamic effort soon after myocardial infarction. *American Heart Journal*, **110**, 542-545; 1985.

95. Dossa, A., LaRaia, J.P., and Clifford, J. Effects of low intensity strength training in elderly patients with congestive heart failure due to ischemic cardiomyopathy. *Cardiopulmonary Physical Therapy Journal*, **4**, 12; 1993 (abstract).

96. Braith, R.W., Limacher, M.C., Leggett, S.H., and Pollock, M.L. Skeletal muscle strength in heart transplant recipients. *Journal of Heart and Lung Transplantation*, **12**, 1018-1023; 1993.

97. Painter, P., and Tomlanavich, S. Organ transplantation: a second chance at fitness. *Your Patient and Fitness*, **7**, 6-17; 1993.

98. Frederickson, L. *Confronting mitral valve prolapse syndrome*. San Marcos, CA: Avant Books; 1988.

99. Hiatt, W.R., Wolfel, E.E., Meier, R.H., and Regensteiner, J.G. Superiority of treadmill walking exercise versus strength training for patients with peripheral vascular disease. *Circulation*, **90**, 1866-1874; 1994.

100. Pollock, M.L., and Wilmore, J.H. *Exercise in health and disease—evaluation and prescription for prevention and rehabilitation*. Orlando, FL: Saunders; 1990.

101. American College of Sports Medicine. The recommended quantity and quality of exercise for developing and maintaining cardiorespiratory and muscular fitness in healthy adults. *Medicine and Science in Sports and Exercise*, **22**, 265-274; 1990.

102. Graves, J.E., Pollock, M.L., Jones, A.E., Colvin, A.B., and Leggett, S.H. Specificity of limited range of motion variable resistance training. *Medicine and Science in Sports and Exercise*, **21**, 84-89; 1989.

103. Pollock, M.L., Carroll, J.F., Graves, J.E., Leggett, S.H., Braith, R.W., Limacher, M., and Hagberg, J. Injuries and adherence to walk/jog and resistance training programs in the elderly. *Medicine and Science in Sports and Exercise*, **23**, 1194-1200; 1991.

104. Starkey, D.B., Pollock, M.L., Ishida, Y., Welsch, M.A., Brechue, W.F., Graves, J.E., and Feigenbaum, M.S. Effect of resistive training volume on strength and muscle thickness. *Medicine and Science in Sports and Exercise*, **28**, 1311-1320; 1996.

105. Shaw, C.E., McCully, K.K., and Posner, J.D. Injuries during the one repetition maximum assessment in the elderly. *Journal of Cardiopulmonary Rehabilitation*, **15**, 283-287; 1995.

106. Gordon, N.F., Kohl, H.W., Pollock, M.L., Vaandrager, H., Gibbons, L.W., and Blair, S.N. Cardiovascular safety of maximal strength testing in healthy adults. *American Journal of Cardiology,* **76**, 851-853; 1995.

107. Gleeson, P.B., Protas, E.J., LeBlanc, A.D., Schneider, V.S., and Evans, H.J. Effects of weight-lifting on the bone mineral density in premenopausal women. *Journal of Bone Mineral Research,* **5**, 153-158; 1990.

108. Heinrich, C.H., Going, S.B., Pamenter, R.W., Perry, C.D., Boyden, T.W., and Lohman, T.G. Bone mineral content of cyclically menstruating female resistance and endurance trained athletes. *Medicine and Science in Sports and Exercise,* **22**, 558-563; 1990.

109. Gordon, N.F., Kohl, H.W., Villegas, J.A., Pickett, K.P., Vaandrager, H., and Duncan, J.J. Effect of rest interval duration on cardiorespiratory responses to hydraulic resistance circuit training. *Journal of Cardiopulmonary Rehabilitation,* **9**, 325-330; 1989.

110. Kraemer, W.J., Noble, B.J., and Clark, M.J. Physiologic responses to heavy-resistance exercise with very short rest periods. *International Journal of Sports Medicine,* **8**, 247-252; 1987.

111. Haennel, R.G., Koon-Kang, T., Quinney, H.A., and Kappagoda, C.T. Effects of hydraulic circuit training on cardiovascular function. *Medicine and Science in Sports and Exercise,* **21**, 605-612; 1989.

112. American College of Cardiology. Recommendations of the American College of Cardiology on cardiovascular rehabilitation. *Journal of the American College of Cardiology,* **7**, 451-453; 1990.

113. Borg, G. Psychophysical basis of perceived exertion. *Medicine and Science in Sports and Exercise,* **14**, 377-381; 1982.

114. Herbert, D.L., and Herbert, W.G. *Legal aspects of preventive, rehabilitative and recreational exercise programs* (3rd ed.). Canton, OH: Professional Reports Corporation; 1993.

115. Sol, N., and Foster, C. *ACSM's health/fitness facility standards and guidelines.* Champaign, IL: Human Kinetics; 1992.

Chapter 3

Aquatics Programming in Cardiac Rehabilitation

John P. Porcari, PhD

Bo Fernhall, PhD

Philip K. Wilson, EdD

E xercise in the water has been popular for many years, particularly for improving fitness in populations with special needs. We see this in special programs for individuals with obesity, orthopedic conditions, neuromuscular and arthritic problems, or low levels of fitness (1-3). The primary reasons for the popularity of water-based exercise with these populations are that the buoyancy afforded by the water reduces lower-joint stress and that the resistance created by moving one's limbs through the water provides a stimulus for muscular development (4, 5).

Safety of Water Exercise in Cardiac Rehabilitation

More recently, water-based activities have also become popular in cardiac rehabilitation programs. However, recommending water exercise for patients with coronary heart disease (CHD) has been controversial. Concerns have arisen because some of the physiological changes that accompany immersion could theoretically jeopardize a diseased myocardium. These include possible increases in left ventricular stress, increases in angina, and the possibility of increased ventricular irritability with cold water immersion (6-9). Table 3.1 provides a summary of possible problems associated with immersion for patients with cardiovascular disease. From a practical standpoint, patient monitoring, exercise prescription, and emergency precautions are more complicated during exercise in the water.

Most concerns about the safety and appropriateness of water exercise for patients with CHD are based on extrapolation of data from populations without CHD, and it appears that many myths have been created. It is important to make an informed decision about using water-based exercise in cardiac rehabilitation. Therefore, in this chapter we will provide an overview of the physiological responses to immersion and

Table 3.1   A Summary of Possible Problems Associated With Water Exercise in Cardiac Patients

Possible problem	Physiological change	Possible clinical outcome
• Increased central blood volume	↑ stroke volume ↑ cardiac output ↓ heart rate ↑ L V volume	↑ LV wall stress ↑ angina ↑ ST depression
• Cold water exposure	↓ heart rate ↑ $PaCO_2$	↑ venticular irritability ↑ arrhythmias

Practical concerns:
- Heart rate — problems with exercise prescription
- Monitoring — problems with ECG and BP monitoring
- Safety — emergency procedures become more complicated

exercise in water in patients with and without CHD. We will also present specific examples of water-based programs and exercise prescription guidelines.

Effects of Immersion at Rest

Water immersion produces a drop in resting heart rate, known as the diving reflex, in both patients with CHD and those without (7, 10-14). This decrease is independent of beta blockade (7, 14), as a similar decrease is seen in patients who are taking beta blockers and in those not taking them (see fig. 3.1). However, the decrease in heart rate becomes more exaggerated with increasing depth of immersion (13) and with colder water temperatures (12, 15), particularly at water temperatures below 25°C. Thus, resting heart rate consistently drops upon water entry in most pool or beach settings, regardless of CHD status.

Immersion causes an increase in hydrostatic pressure that in turn increases both stroke volume and cardiac output at rest (12, 13, 15-18). These changes occur in patients with and without CHD. However, because of lower peripheral resistance, total cardiac work is not different between sitting on land and sitting immersed in water (6, 14, 19). Furthermore, immersion reduces vital capacity and may reduce gas exchange, but has no effect on oxygen uptake (17, 20-22). Thus, despite changes in cardiovascular and pulmonary variables, immersion in thermoneutral water does not increase left ventricular stress or overall metabolism at rest.

Diving in cold water has been shown to produce ventricular arrhythmias in both men and women without CHD (23-25). This seems to be related to both the depth of diving and the water temperature. It has been suggested that the diving reflex may be exaggerated in some individuals, and this may have been related to sudden death due to an extreme bradycardiac response in at least one individual (25, 26). The mechanism of the increased rate of arrhythmias may be related to a decrease in the partial

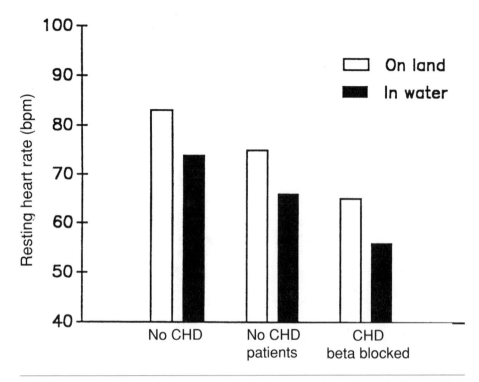

Figure 3.1   The effect of immersion on resting heart rate in patients with and without CHD. Notice that for the CHD patients, beta blockade did not change the immersion effect.

pressure of carbon dioxide with immersion in cold water, producing higher ventricular irritability (9).

During cardiac rehabilitation, occasional ectopic beats may occur upon water entry (27), but nothing untoward that would prevent safe exercise in the water has been reported. We have observed that some patients may experience slight anginal episodes on water entry but that these quickly disappear while they are resting in the water. Furthermore, the development of angina on water entry is very unusual and does not occur in most patients.

Exercise Responses During Immersion Responses

In patients without CHD, swimming produces markedly lower maximal oxygen uptake ($\dot{V}O_2$max) (see fig. 3.2) and maximal heart rates (see fig. 3.3) than either treadmill or cycling exercise on land (28-30). This has been attributed to the effects of immersion, but may also be related to body position and muscle mass. Since swimming uses less muscle mass than walking or running, maximal responses would be expected to be lower, with differences in maximal heart rate to be further exacerbated by immersion.

Maximal swimming in patients with CHD also produces markedly lower $\dot{V}O_2$max values than treadmill testing on land (31, 32) (see fig. 3.2); this is similar to what

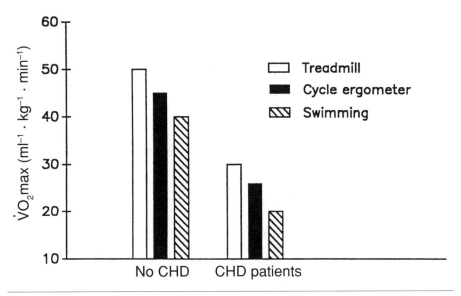

Figure 3.2   Maximal oxygen uptake ($\dot{V}O_2$max) during three different types of exercise for individuals with and without CHD. Note that all subjects have lower $\dot{V}O_2$max when swimming and that treadmill exercise yields the highest values.

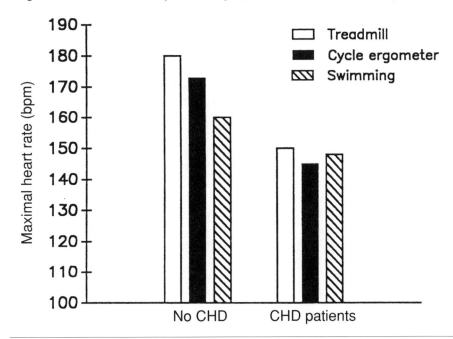

Figure 3.3   Maximal heart rate during three different types of exercise for individuals with and without CHD. Note that for persons without CHD the maximal heart rate is highest for treadmill testing and lowest for swimming. However, for CHD patients, there is essentially no difference in maximal heart rate between exercise modes.

occurs in persons without CHD. In contrast to patients without CHD, however, CHD patients exhibit no difference in maximal heart rate between swimming, cycling, and running (7, 27, 31, 32) (see fig. 3.3). In persons without CHD, maximal heart rates are usually 10-20% lower during swimming. It has been suggested that CHD patients have similar heart rates for swimming and treadmill testing because they are less limited by cardiac symptoms during swimming (7, 27).

The lower $\dot{V}O_2$max during swimming in patients with CHD is probably a result of a lower cardiac output, despite a similar maximal heart rate (7). Maximal cardiac output has been shown to be 25% lower during swimming in cardiac patients—a response considerably different from that of their peers without CHD (7). The reason for the lower cardiac output is that stroke volume does not change from rest to exercise during swimming in CHD patients (7). Thus, the increase in cardiac output during swimming is entirely dependent on the increase in heart rate.

It is also possible that a higher peripheral resistance, as a result of arm activity, lowers the stroke volume because of limitations to venous return. However, recent data suggest that peripheral resistance is lower in the water than during land exercise (14). Instead, it has been suggested that preload is already maximal as a result of immersion and that patients with CHD do not have the ability to further increase preload in response to exercise (18). Therefore, their ability to increase stroke volume through the Frank-Starling mechanism would be limited. This is possibly attributable to reduced ventricular compliance during diastole and/or abnormal systolic function (18).

During submaximal exercise in patients without CHD, exercise heart rates are lower at the same $\dot{V}O_2$ during swimming than during treadmill exercise (see fig. 3.4b), showing a persistent effect of the diving reflex (28, 29). This response is further exaggerated during cold water swimming. In CHD patients, heart rate is reduced at rest in the water but not during swim exercise (7, 14, 27, 31, 32); this is different from what occurs in their peers without CHD. In fact, a "cross-over" occurs at very low levels of exercise, between 30% and 40% of $\dot{V}O_2$max (see fig. 3.4a). Swimming above this intensity does not produce depressed heart rates, suggesting that the "diving reflex" is not operative during swimming in CHD patients. Similar results have also been shown during water cycling (14, 18).

Since maximal heart rate does not differ between water and land exercise in patients with CHD, and the diving reflex is not operative at submaximal exercise, the relative relationship between $\dot{V}O_2$ and heart rate is the same during water and land exercise. This means that water exercise can be accurately prescribed from exercise testing on land (7, 31-33). In fact, it was found that exercise prescriptions for water exercise (water aerobics) and swimming could be accurately determined from either treadmill or cycle ergometer testing, but that data from arm ergometry did not accurately prescribe exercise intensity at levels above 60% of maximum (33). Thus, arm ergometry should not be used to generate exercise prescriptions for water exercise, including swimming. Although tethered swimming yields accurate test results for CHD patients, it is not a feasible method of testing in most situations (31, 32). Data also suggest that water running can be accurately prescribed from treadmill test data in patients with CHD (4, 5, 34, 35).

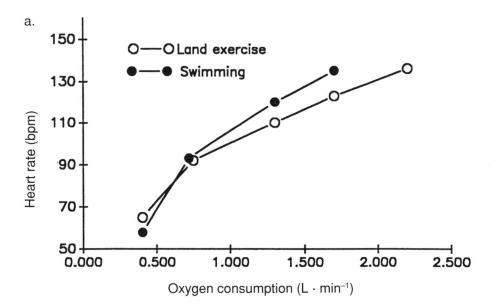

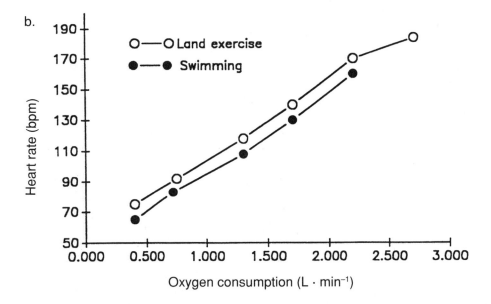

Figure 3.4   A comparison of the HR/$\dot{V}O_2$ relationship in individuals with and without CHD, during swimming and land exercise. Note that in CHD patients (a), maximal heart rate is similar between water and land exercise and that HR is higher at the same $\dot{V}O_2$ during water exercise. In normal populations without CHD (b), HR during swimming is consistently below HR on land at the same $\dot{V}O_2$, and maximal heart rate is higher on land than in the water.

It is important to note that swimming may not be an appropriate mode of exercise for many CHD patients. Even easy, comfortable swimming yields heart rates between 85% and 90% of maximum, which may be too high for many individuals (27, 33, 36). Both the heart rate and $\dot{V}O_2$ generated during swimming are closely tied to swimming skill. Small increases in swimming speed will produce large changes in both heart rate and $\dot{V}O_2$ in some individuals but will have little effect on others (27). Furthermore, the rating of perceived exertion (RPE) is not a reliable indicator of exercise intensity during swimming (33). Therefore, poorly skilled swimmers with CHD should probably avoid this form of exercise. Since water aerobics allows for better flexibility and control over heart rate, and does not require breath-holding or facial immersion, it can easily be substituted for swimming.

Clinical Exercise Responses During Immersion

Breath-hold diving may produce cardiac arrhythmias, and cold water diving could increase ventricular irritability in individuals without CHD (23-25). Because cold air during the winter months can be angina provoking in CHD patients, and because some CHD patients may experience angina upon water entry, similar concerns have been raised for swimming. Swimming with facial immersion has been of special concern because of the possible contribution of the cold pressor response (37).

Very little research has been conducted on the ECG responses to swimming in patients with CHD. In general, patients who show ST-segment displacement during their stress test also show ST-segment displacement during swimming (14). The ST-segment changes also occur at similar heart rates for both land and water exercise, suggesting little difference in the ST-segment response to water and land-based exercise. Furthermore, ST-segment changes during swimming in cool (25 °C) and cold water (18 °C) do not differ (27). However, while five subjects experienced angina when exercising on land, only two had angina with warm water exercise, and only one had angina with cold water exercise (27). These data suggest that water exercise may mask anginal symptoms even in the presence of significant ST-segment depression. This response may be temperature dependent, but it is important to remember that the number of subjects studied was very small, making it difficult to draw substantive conclusions.

More recent research has evaluated the incidence of ST-segment displacement and arrhythmias during regular cardiac rehabilitation sessions conducted on land or in the water (8, 33, 38, 39). Whether the ECG was monitored through a quick check with a defibrillator (38) or through continuous telemetry (8, 33, 39), there was no increase in ECG changes with water exercise, although one study found that asymptomatic ST-segment depression (1 mm) did occur at lower heart rates in the water (39). During these actual cardiac rehabilitation sessions there was also no difference in anginal incidence between water and land-based exercise, and angina occurred at similar heart rates. Thus, the information to date indicates that water exercise in warm or cool water does not increase ECG signs or clinical symptoms in CHD patients, but the effect of very cold water (less than 16 °C) has not been investigated.

Summary

Immersion causes a decrease in resting heart rate in CHD patients. Unlike what occurs in individuals without CHD, this decrease at rest does not persist throughout exercise. Maximal heart rate is similar between land and water exercise, but $\dot{V}O_2$max is higher on land. Therefore, heart rate is higher at the same submaximal level of $\dot{V}O_2$ during water exercise. Cardiac output is lower during swimming, despite similar or higher heart rates, because of much lower stroke volumes. In fact, stroke volume does not increase significantly from resting values during exercise in the water, probably because of possible reductions in ventricular compliance during diastole and/or abnormal systolic function.

The relationship between %HRmax and %$\dot{V}O_2$max is similar between water and land exercise in CHD patients. This means that one can appropriately prescribe exercise intensity from conventional exercise testing except for arm ergometry. However, because heart rate during swimming is highly dependent on swimming skill, this activity must be monitored closely, and water aerobics may need to be substituted for swimming with many CHD patients.

There is no evidence to suggest that water exercise increases the risk of untoward events in CHD patients as long as the water temperature is moderate. No research has shown any increases in ECG signs or in clinical symptoms suggestive of ischemia during water exercise. Thus, water exercise appears to be a safe alternative to conventional cardiac rehabilitation programs.

Patient Selection

Water exercise appears to be most beneficial for low- to moderate-risk cardiac patients who either like to swim or have orthopedic or arthritic problems that may be aggravated by traditional land-based exercise modalities (i.e., walking or cycling). Water exercise is also of particular benefit in those individuals limited by peripheral vascular disease, particularly if the water temperature is in the range of 30-33 °C (86-92 °F). The warmer water facilitates peripheral vasodilation, and the added buoyancy afforded by the water reduces lower-limb stress, allowing for longer exercise durations (40).

On the basis of current knowledge, it is probably best to restrict exercise in the water to low- and moderate-risk patients because of difficulties in monitoring patients and carrying out emergency protocols in the pool. Additionally, there are no data available on the hemodynamic responses of high-risk patients to immersion or exercise in the water. Table 3.2 lists a number of characteristics and factors that would place patients in a "high-risk" category or would identify those individuals at high risk for developing complications during exercise training. This list has been adapted from a review of the recommendations presented by the American College of Physicians (41), the American College of Cardiology (42), and the American Association of Cardiovascular and Pulmonary Rehabilitation (43). It should be noted that we have not included absolute guidelines delimiting patients based on functional capacity (maximal METs). We prefer to evaluate patients on an individual basis, and in fact have cardiac patients utilizing the pool with aerobic capacities ranging from 5 to 17 METs.

Exercise Prescription Considerations

When one is prescribing exercise in the water, it is necessary to consider a number of practical factors. Among these are the temperature of the water and the frequency, intensity, and duration of exercise.

Water Temperature

The water temperature recommended for cardiac rehabilitation programs varies, ranging from 26 to 33 °C (80-92 °F) (35, 44). Water at the lower end of this range is best for heat dissipation during exercise, whereas temperatures at the upper end are considered more comfortable for the majority of patients. If the majority of your patients have orthopedic problems, arthritis, or peripheral vascular disease, the upper end of the recommended range is most desirable. In many situations it is not possible to control the pool temperature (e.g., at a YMCA or in a university setting). Therefore it should be emphasized that any of the temperatures within the recommended range are acceptable and should not result in adverse clinical signs or symptoms; patient comfort is the best guide. However, patients who exercise at high intensities for longer than 20 minutes in the upper end of this range may find it uncomfortable. The only absolute contraindication is that the temperature shouldn't be below 15 °C (60 °F), since studies have not been conducted on cardiac patients in water below this temperature.

Exercise Intensity

Exercise intensity should be prescribed based on the American College of Sports Medicine guidelines and may range from 40% to 85% of functional capacity depending on the age and capabilities of individual patients (40). We typically start uncom-

Table 3.2   Characteristics of Patients That Place Them in a High-Risk Category or at High Risk for Developing Complications During Exercise Training

1. Severely depressed left ventricular function (EF < 30%)
2. Resting complex ventricular ectopy
3. Appearance of or increasing ventricular ectopy with exercise
4. Severe CAD and marked exercise-induced myocardial ischemia (>2 mm ST depression)
5. A drop in systolic blood pressure with exercise or failure of the blood pressure to rise from resting values with the onset of exercise
6. Being a survivor of sudden cardiac death
7. Being a survivor of myocardial infarction complicated by congestive heart failure, cardiogenic shock, and/or serious ventricular arrhythmias
8. Inability to self-monitor exercise HR because of physical or intellectual impairment

plicated patients at 50-60% of maximal capacity and progress upward from there. As mentioned earlier, exercise heart rates can be accurately prescribed from treadmill or cycle ergometer tests (7, 33, 34). Keep in mind that RPE may not be a good indicator of exercise intensity during exercise in the water (35) (i.e., RPE is lower at any given heart rate), and note especially the need for accurate monitoring of exercise pulse rates, particularly in patients who have rate-dependent ischemia, arrhythmias, etc. Additionally, anginal symptoms may be masked in the water (32), so patients may be without their own best warning signal of impending problems.

Frequency and Duration of Exercise

Once again, recommendations about frequency and duration should be consistent with American College of Sports Medicine guidelines (40). Most programs, ours included, are conducted 3 days per week. Additionally, we advise patients to try to exercise another 1-2 days per week on their own by incorporating walking or stationary cycling at home. These recommendations are also consistent with the latest information suggesting that most adults should get at least 30 minutes of moderate-intensity physical activity most days of the week in order to positively affect their health (45). While these recommendations were not specifically targeting cardiac patients per se, we feel that this advice can be extended to them. Also, since many cardiac patients are trying to control body weight and body fat, exercising 4-5 days per week increases total caloric expenditure and should promote better control of body composition.

The aerobic portion of each water exercise period should last at least 20-30 minutes. In that period of time, our typical patient swims an average of 1,000 yards (range of 500-2,000 yards) depending upon the stroke. Patients who engage solely in water walking typically walk between 400 and 700 yards per workout.

Warm-Up and Cool-Down

Before the beginning of any exercise bout, a proper warm-up is essential. For cardiac patients this may be even more true, since water entry has been shown to cause angina in some patients. We have all patients perform 3-5 minutes of stretching and light calisthenics on the pool deck before entering the water. Exercises are performed for the neck, shoulders, triceps, trunk, groin, hamstrings, and calf. We also urge a gradual entry into the pool down the ladder.

Cool-down exercises are usually conducted in the water and consist of 3-5 minutes of free-standing and wall stretches. We have found that it is easier and more comfortable for participants to do the cool-down in the water, since once people leave the water, the air is invariably colder than the water and they become easily chilled. Ideally we like participants to get their pulse rates below 100 before exiting the pool.

Other Programming Considerations

When one deals with cardiac patients, exercise in a water environment poses other practical problems that need to be considered and addressed. These include monitoring patient responses to exercise and handling emergency situations if they arise.

Patient Monitoring

In the initial stages of the program, frequent blood pressure and heart rate checks should be required. As patients become more comfortable with exercising in the water, and you are assured that they are responding appropriately, you can decrease the frequency of monitoring. Monitoring of the exercise ECG is preferable during the early stages of rehabilitation (39); however, most facilities do not have the specialized telemetry equipment necessary to monitor patients in the water. Periodic monitoring with "quick-look" paddles is another alternative, but with this method there is a high chance that arrhythmias may go undetected (38). If a patient is having palpable rhythm problems, then a quick-look scan is recommended as a way of trying to determine the nature of the rhythm disturbance. Blood pressure measurements can similarly be made poolside.

Emergency Procedures

Well-planned emergency procedures must be in place for all parts of your cardiac rehabilitation program and must be practiced on a regular basis. In the pool this is even more crucial. Because of the difficulties of conducting a code situation in a water environment, a minimum of two staff members should be present at all times.

In the event of an emergency, the patient should be removed from the water as quickly as possible. A drainboard and extra towels should always be immediately available in case defibrillation becomes necessary. In such an event, the patient should be dried off completely and placed on the drainboard before any attempt at defibrillating is made. Special care should be taken to ensure that the chest is completely dry, as "arcing" of the electrical current may occur if any moisture is present. Extreme care should be taken that the staff person performing the resuscitation not be standing or kneeling in water, and ideally that person should be wearing rubber-soled shoes.

Aquatic Activities

A wide variety of exercise activities can be prescribed in the water, and the intensity of these activities can vary from very low to extremely high. Unfortunately, there are limited data on the actual energy cost of most water activities, especially in cardiac patients. Therefore, many of our suggestions are based upon data from healthy adults, intuition, and our experience.

Water Walking

Walking in the water is probably the safest exercise and the easiest exercise to control from an intensity viewpoint. The energy cost is determined primarily by the depth of the water, the walking speed, and the degree of arm involvement. The greatest energy cost during water walking can be attained in a water depth between the knees and midthigh (28). Going deeper than this actually decreases energy cost, as the buoyant forces afforded by the water offset the increased resistance that comes from having water coverage over a greater body surface area. Therefore, patients need to be aware that if they walk in deeper water, energy cost is going to be lower.

Quite obviously the energy cost and resultant intensity increase as the speed of walking increases. Energy cost is a linear function of speed up to approximately 53.6 m × min^{-1} (2 mph) and is curvilinear thereafter (28). It is important to note, however, that this research was conducted on an underwater treadmill and that most cardiac patients cannot walk fast enough in a regular pool to attain these speeds; therefore energy cost for these individuals will remain a linear function of walking speed.

Another way to increase exercise intensity is to involve the arms during walking. The arms can be used in a simulated swimming motion either above (front crawl) or below (breast stroke) the surface of the water. Little data are available on the added energy cost of this activity; however, Fernhall et al. (33) have shown that by walking/ jogging with simultaneous arm movement, patients can easily elicit intensities of 80% HRmax. Another added benefit of involving arm movement is to condition and strengthen the upper body and ensure a total-body workout.

In our experience, patients need to be constantly reminded to push themselves when walking in the water. Many patients find it more enjoyable to walk slowly and social- ize than to seriously pursue their exercise goals.

Swimnastics or Water Aerobics

The next level of intensity is probably afforded by upright water exercise, or what is commonly referred to as "swimnastics" or water aerobics. These activities are usually conducted in a group setting, but the same movements can be performed individually. The added benefit of performing these activities in a group setting is the social atmo- sphere and the camaraderie that quickly develops among program participants, in many cases enhancing exercise adherence.

Swimnastics is essentially aerobic dance conducted in the water. A typical class usually involves a 5-10-minute warm-up, 15-20 minutes of aerobic arm and leg move- ments conducted singly or in combination, 10 minutes of resistive arm and leg exer- cises, and a 5-minute cool-down. The resistive movements are usually conducted using commercially available water dumbbells, floats, or paddles. We have found milk jugs to be an inexpensive alternative, especially since they can be filled with water to varying degrees and used as weights to condition the arms and shoulders.

Many water aerobics classes for younger populations also include exercise in the deeper (over the head) sections of the pool, requiring individuals to tread water to keep themselves afloat and maintain an upright body position. In our experience this activity can promote a good deal of breath-holding and isometric activity, which should be avoided in a cardiac population.

One new activity we have incorporated into our swimnastics program is aqua-step- ping, which is step aerobics in the water. Exercises using the weighted steps (which are virtually identical to steps used on land) have been added to all of our classes and again have proven to add variety and increase enjoyment for participants. Aqua-steps are now commercially available from most major aquatics suppliers.

Swimming

Participants can use a variety of swimming strokes, including the modified back- stroke, breast stroke, side stroke, and the front crawl. In the modified back stroke, the arms are brought up alongside the body to a position perpendicular to the long axis of the torso, not windmilled overhead as in a competitive backstroke. Unfortunately, the only data available on the energy requirements of these strokes are on competitive swimmers (46), and this information is probably not applicable to the actual energy costs for cardiac patients using these strokes.

For the modified backstroke, side stroke, and breast stroke, the intensity can be fairly well controlled and is within reach of most cardiac patients. The energy cost of the front crawl, however, can vary tremendously with the efficiency of the swimmer. Several authors (32, 35, 36) recommend that cardiac patients not use the front crawl, since exercise intensity can easily exceed 80-85% of HRmax. In our experience, most people, cardiac patients included, are not very efficient swimmers. However, if given proper instruction in stroke mechanics, they can become much more efficient, and can do the front crawl. Frequently, patients will alternate between the front crawl and one of the other strokes.

One of the factors that most affect the energy requirements of the front crawl is head position. Good swimmers have their face immersed in the water and turn their head to the side to breathe. Poor swimmers have their head completely out of the water at all times. Supporting the head in this fashion greatly increases swimming resistance and adds to the energy cost of performing the stroke. Several years ago a unique solution was suggested by one of our participants—the use of a snorkel. Since then, several of our patients have used a snorkel while doing the front crawl (see fig. 3.5), eliminating the need to work so hard to keep the head up. In our experience this has worked extremely well. One must realize, however, that potential problems may exist with facial immersion (37); in addition, the snorkel makes it impossible to see a patient's face in the event of problems, and this may delay recognition of abnormal signs and symptoms.

While we don't specifically test to assess swimming skill or to determine how patients respond to the various swimming strokes, such testing is easy to do and may provide a basis for allowing patients to advance to the more difficult strokes. In this case, monitoring of exercise heart rates would be the best guide to assure that patients are staying within their individual exercise prescriptions.

Water Volleyball

Another fun alternative for exercising in the water is water volleyball. Water volleyball is played in the shallow end of the pool with the water at approximately waist to nipple level. Rules modifications that we use include allowing an unlimited number of hits on each side and allowing a player to hit the ball more than once in succession. While water volleyball should not replace the aerobic portion of a person's exercise session (we require all participants to exercise aerobically for at least 20-30 minutes before they play volleyball), it has proven to be an extremely popular way to end each day (see fig. 3.6).

Inner-Tube Games

In addition to water volleyball, we have found that inner-tube basketball and inner-tube water polo are extremely popular with participants. Not only are they pleasant

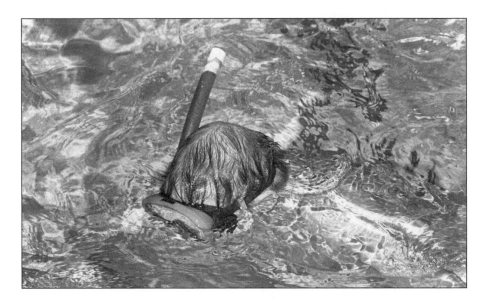

Figure 3.5 The energy cost of performing the front crawl can be greatly affected by individual skill level, and many inefficient swimmers struggle to breathe by lifting their heads out of the water. We have found that allowing people to use a snorkel while swimming enables them to perform the front crawl and still stay within their prescribed target heart rates.

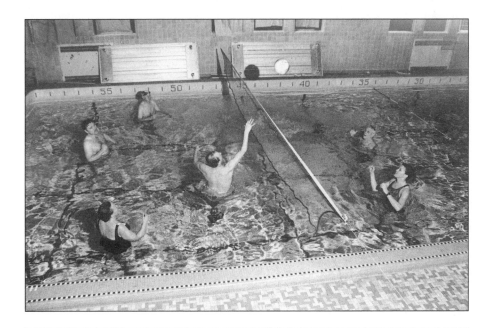

Figure 3.6 Water volleyball has proven to be a popular activity that adds variety to a workout.

activities, but they are not dependent on swimming ability, so everyone can enjoy them. Additionally, they provide a water "game" alternative if the pool does not have a shallow end where people can easily do water aerobics or play water volleyball. Inner tubes can be purchased at any service station; however, most programs have a resourceful participant or two who could procure used tubes free of charge and patch them as need be.

Conclusions

Water provides an excellent medium for exercising cardiac patients, especially those with arthritic or orthopedic problems, since the buoyancy afforded by the water limits the amount of joint stress and allows exercise duration to be increased. A variety of exercise options have been shown to be of sufficient intensity for training, including water walking, swimnastics or water aerobics, and a number of swimming strokes. One must use caution when prescribing the various swimming strokes, however, since skill level of the individual can greatly affect energy cost. Additionally, exercise sessions can be augmented with a variety of water games, such as water volleyball or inner-tube games, for added enjoyment. All sessions should be preceded by a warm-up session, and pool entry should be gradual. Exercise intensity can be prescribed using standard techniques from both treadmill and cycle ergometer testing data. The safety of exercising in the water has been shown to be similar to that of other forms of exercise. However, because of the logistical problems associated with handling emergencies in the water, emergency protocols must be in place and must be practiced regularly. Although to our knowledge there are no training studies that have investigated the effects of water exercise or swimming in patients with CHD, it can be presumed that training benefits would be comparable to those seen with land-based exercise if training intensity and frequency are matched.

References

1. Fisher, S.V., and Gullickson, G. Energy cost of ambulation in health and disease: a literature review. *Archives of Physical Medicine and Rehabilitation,* **59**, 124-133; 1979.
2. Guber, R.S. Spa therapy in cardiovascular rehabilitation. Proceedings of Fourth World Congress, International Rehabilitation Medical Association, San Juan, Puerto Rico; 1982: p. 124.
3. Lavoie, J.M., and Montpetit, R.R. Applied physiology of swimming. *Sports Medicine,* **3**, 165-189; 1986.
4. Svedenhag, J., and Segar, J. Running on land and in water: comparative exercise physiology. *Medicine and Science in Sports and Exercise,* **24**, 1155-1160; 1992.
5. Wilder, R.P., Brennan, D., and Schotte, D.E. A standard measure for exercise prescription for aqua running. *American Journal of Sports Medicine,* **21**, 45-48; 1993.

6. Arborelius, M., Balldin, U., Lilja, B., and Lundgren, C.E.G. Hemodynamic changes in man during immersion with the head above water. *Aerospace Medicine,* **43**, 592-598; 1972.

7. Heigenhauser, G.F., Boulet, D., Miller, B., and Faulkner, J.A. Cardiac output of post-myocardial infarction patients during swimming and cycling. *Medicine and Science in Sports,* **9**, 143-147; 1977.

8. Fernhall, B., Congdon, K., and Manfredi, T. ECG response to water and land based exercise in patients with cardiovascular disease. *Journal of Cardiopulmonary Rehabilitation,* **10**, 5-11; 1990.

9. DeMerlier, K. Value of swimming in cardiac rehabilitation and internal medicine. In: Hollander, A.P., Itnijong, P.A., deGroot, G., eds. *Biomechanics and medicine in swimming, International Series on Sport Sciences.* Champaign, IL: Human Kinetics; 1983:pp. 17-27.

10. Haffor, A.S.A., Mohler, J.G., and Harrison, A.C. Effects of water immersion on cardiac output of lean and fat male subjects at rest and during exercise. *Aviation, Space, and Environmental Medicine,* **62**, 123-127; 1991.

11. Dressendorfer, R.H., Morlock, J.F., Baker, D.G., and Hong, S.K. Effects of head-out water immersion on cardiorespiratory responses to maximal exercise. *Undersea Biomedicine Research,* **3**, 177-187; 1976.

12. Choukroun, M.L., and Varene, P. Adjustments in oxygen transport during head-out immersion in water at different temperatures. *Journal of Applied Physiology,* **68**, 1475-1480; 1990.

13. Risch, W.D., Koubenec, H.J., Beckman, U., Lange, S., and Gauer, O.H. The effect of graded immersion on heart volume, venous pressure, pulmonary blood distribution, and heart rate in man. *Pfluger's Archives,* **374**, 115-118; 1978.

14. McMurray, R.G., Fieselman, C.C., Avery, K.E., and Sheps, D.S. Exercise hemodynamics in water and on land in patients with coronary heart disease. *Journal of Cardiopulmonary Rehabilitation,* **8**, 69-75; 1988.

15. McArdle, W.D., Magel, J.R., Lesmes, G.R., and Pechar, G.S. Metabolic and cardiovascular adjustment to work in air and water at 18, 25, and 33C. *Journal of Applied Physiology,* **40**, 85-90; 1976.

16. Begin, R., Epstein, M., Sackner, M.A., Levinson, R., Dougherty, R., and Duncan, D. Effects of water immersion to the neck on pulmonary circulation and tissue volume in man. *Journal of Applied Physiology,* **40**, 293-299; 1976.

17. Farhi, L.E., and Linnarson, D. Cardiopulmonary readjustments during graded immersion in water at 35C. *Respiration Physiology,* **30**, 35-50; 1977.

18. Hanna, R., Sheldahl, L.M., and Tristani, F.E. Effect of enhanced preload with head-out immersion on exercise response in men with healed myocardial infarction. *American Journal of Cardiology,* **71**, 1041-1044; 1993.

19. Lin, Y.C. Circulatory functions during immersion and breath-hold dives in humans. *Undersea Biomedicine Research,* **11**, 123-138; 1984.

20. Arborelius, M., Balldin, U., Lilja, B., and Lundgren, C.E.G. Regional lung function in man during immersion with the head above water. *Aerospace Medicine,* **43**, 701-707; 1972.

21. Cohen, R., Bell, W.H., Saltzman, H.A., and Kylstra, J.A. Alveolo-arterial oxy-

gen pressure difference in man immersed up to the neck in water. *Journal of Applied Physiology,* **30**, 720-723; 1971.

22. Prefaut, C., Ramonatxo, M., Boyer, Q., and Chardon, G. Human gas exchange during water immersion. *Respiration Physiology,* **34**, 307-319; 1978.

23. Hong, S.K., and Rahn, H. The diving women of Korea and Japan. *Scientific American,* **216**, 34-43; 1967.

24. Jung, K., and Stolle, W. Behavior of heart rate and incidence of arrhythmia in swimming and diving. *Biotelemetry and Patient Monitor,* **8**, 228-239; 1981.

25. Lin, Y.C. Applied physiology of diving. *Sports Medicine,* **5**, 41-56; 1988.

26. Wolf, S. The bradycardia of the dive reflex: a possible mechanism of sudden death. *Transcripts of the American Clinical and Climatological Association,* **76**, 142-200; 1964.

27. Magder, S., Linnarson, D., and Gullstrand, L. The effect of swimming on patients with ischemic heart disease. *Circulation,* **63**, 979-986; 1981.

28. Holmer, I. Physiology of swimming. *Acta Physiologica Scandinavica,* **407**(Suppl.):1-55; 1974.

29. Nadel, E.R., Holmer, I., Berg, V., Astrand, P.O., and Stolwijk, J.A. Energy exchange in swimming man. *Journal of Applied Physiology,* **36**, 465-571; 1974.

30. Avellini, B.A., Shapiro, Y., and Pandolf, K. Cardio-respiratory physical training in water and on land. *Journal of Applied Physiology,* **50**, 255-263; 1983.

31. Thompson, D.L., Boone, W.T., and Miller, H.S. Comparison of treadmill exercise and tethered swimming to determine validity of exercise prescription. *Journal of Cardiac Rehabilitation,* **2**, 363-372; 1982.

32. Boone, W.T., and Thompson, D.L. Reproducibility of tethered swimming in exercise rehabilitation research. *American Corrective Therapy,* **37**, 23-27; 1983.

33. Fernhall, B., Manfredi, T.G., and Congdon, K. Prescribing water based exercise from treadmill and arm ergometry in cardiac patients. *Medicine and Science in Sports and Exercise,* **24**, 139-143; 1992.

34. Gleim, G.W., and Nicholas, J.A. Metabolic cost and heart rate responses to treadmill walking in water at different depths and temperatures. *American Journal of Sports Medicine,* **17**, 248-252; 1989.

35. Evans, B.W., Cureton, K.J., and Purvis, J.W. Metabolic and circulatory responses to walking and jogging in water. *Research Quarterly,* **49**, 442-449; 1978.

36. Fletcher, G.F., Cantwell, J.D., and Watt, E.W. Oxygen consumption and hemodynamic response of exercise used in training of patients with recent myocardial infarction. *Circulation,* **60**, 140-144; 1979.

37. Rogers, P.J., Bove, A.A., Squires, R.W., and Bailey, K.R. Cardiovascular responses to the cold pressor test in exercise trained and untrained men. *Journal of Cardiopulmonary Rehabilitation,* **8**, 518-524; 1988.

38. Lloyd, A., Thiel, J., Holloman, P., Fletcher, B., and Fletcher, G.F. Water exercise versus land exercise in cardiac patients [abstract]. *Journal of Cardiopulmonary Rehabilitation,* **6**, 434; 1986.

39. Niebauer, J., Hambrecht, R., Hauer, K., Marburger, C., Schoppenthau, M., Kalberer, B., Schlief, G., Kubler, W., and Schuler, G. Identification of patients at risk during swimming by holter monitoring. *American Journal of Cardiology,* **74**, 651-656; 1994.

40. American College of Sports Medicine. *Guidelines for exercise testing and prescription,* 4th ed. Philadelphia: Lea & Febiger; 1991.

41. Health and Public Policy Committee, American College of Physicians. Cardiac rehabilitation services. *Annals Internal Medicine,* **15**, 671-673; 1988.

42. American College of Cardiology. Position statement on cardiac rehabilitation. *Journal of American College. Cardiology,* **7**(2):451-453; 1986.

43. American Association of Cardiovascular and Pulmonary Rehabilitation. *Guidelines for cardiac rehabilitation programs.* Champaign, IL: Human Kinetics; 1991.

44. Koszota, L.E. From sweats to swimsuits: is water exercise the wave of the future? *Physician and Sportsmedicine,* **17**(4):203-206; 1989.

45. Summary statement: Workshop on Physical Activity and Public Health. *Sports Medicine Bulletin,* **28**(4):7; 1993.

46. McArdle, W.D., Katch, F.I., and Katch, V.L. *Exercise physiology: energy, nutrition, and human performance,* 3rd ed. Philadelphia: Lea & Febiger; 1991.

Chapter 4

Games-As-Aerobics: Activities for Cardiac Rehabilitation Programs

Barry A. Franklin, PhD

Karl G. Stoedefalke, PhD

T he beneficial effects of regular physical activity are well documented. Aerobic exercise training decreases the heart rate and blood pressure at rest and at any given submaximal work rate, reducing the demands on the heart. Research has also shown that regular exercise increases the maximal oxygen consumption ($\dot{V}O_2$max) or aerobic capacity. Because this variable normally decreases by about 1% per year after the age of 20, and because an exercise program generally increases the $\dot{V}O_2$max by about 20%, the physically conditioned 60-year-old may achieve the same aerobic fitness level as the inactive 40-year-old. In other words, regular exercise can lead to a 20-year functional rejuvenation (1). Mild to moderate exercise intensities also provide numerous health benefits if the frequency and duration of training are sufficient. These benefits include increased bone density, enhanced glucose tolerance, an improved coronary risk factor profile, and reduced cardiovascular-related mortality (2). Moreover, research suggests that compared with sedentary people, those who exercise are better able to cope with stress and are less likely to suffer from depression and anxiety (3, 4).

While many people can be encouraged to initiate a physical conditioning program, fewer than half maintain long-term adherence (5). The problem? In a word, motivation. The comment, "It's not fun until you stop" is a reaction to exercise heard more often than many fitness instructors would like to admit (6). Unfortunately, the exercise experience for a significant number of cardiac patients is more like unpaid labor than play. As research in exercise adherence indicates, such perceptions are strongly associated with the problem of dropout (7). Therefore it is reasonable to ask, Is there a clear link between enjoyment and exercise adherence? Many times enjoyment comes in the form of variety (8). The saying that "variety is the spice of life" is true also of exercise. Indeed, 9 out of 10 participants polled at the 1980 Ironman Triathlon said they began training for all three activities (i.e., swimming, bicycling, running) because they were no longer challenged by a single event (9).

The type of exercise program has been shown to influence long-term adherence. Regimented calisthenics, when relied on too heavily in a physical conditioning program, readily become monotonous and boring, leading to poor exercise adherence. This notion was substantiated by the high dropout rate (70%) reported by the Federal Aviation Agency in an exercise program involving 1,244 employees (10). Similarly, Massie and Shephard (11) examined the effectiveness of individual aerobic exercise (i.e., one person exercising alone) versus supervised exercise in two groups of middle-aged men over a duration of 28 weeks. The supervised program included a variety of stretching, flexibility, strengthening, and aerobic activities. Despite the encouragement provided by completion of exercise "logs," only 47% of the individualized aerobics program recruits were still active at 28 weeks, compared with 82% of the supervised program participants. Others have also reported good exercise adherence in cardiac exercise programs that incorporated varied, pleasurable activities and group dynamics (12) as opposed to more regimented programs in which a person exercises alone (13). Because home-based exercise rehabilitation and supervised, group programs have shown comparable safety and efficacy (14), it appears that varied outcomes are due primarily to differences in the exercise activities, the staffing, or both, rather than in the physical conditioning setting per se.

Although there are countless articles and texts on the scientific basis of exercise programming and prescription (15), exercise leaders need practical ideas and clearly illustrated pleasurable activities (exercises). The "Games-As-Aerobics" approach provides an ideal complement to a walk-jog or cycle ergometer exercise–training program (16). The approach differs from many standard intervention or rehabilitation programs in that it maximizes the pleasure principle. It is predicated on the belief that people seek activities that provide fun and repeated success as opposed to the regimentation associated with many traditional programs. Stretching and flexibility movements are frequently camouflaged in the form of individual or partner activities, games, and relays. Exercises are modified to incorporate ball passing and other movement skills for variety. Furthermore, game rules are altered to minimize skill and competition and maximize participant success. Fitness leaders may also use hula hoops, medicine balls, jump ropes, elastic bands, parachutes, swimming facilities, progressive resistance devices, and other contemporary exercise equipment to diversify their programs. Through such modifications the exercise leader is better able to emphasize the primary goal of the exercise—enjoyment of the game or activity itself.

This chapter describes and illustrates a number of enjoyable stretching and flexibility movements and aerobic activities that should prove useful to fitness instructors, exercise leaders, and physical educators. Use of these individual and partner stationary and continuous–movement exercises, group activities, and recreational games and relays can help stimulate and maintain interest, enthusiasm, and adherence among adult fitness and cardiac rehabilitation program participants.

INDIVIDUAL STATIONARY EXERCISES

The following individual exercises, using a playground ball (9-inch diameter probably has the greatest utility) or volleyball, are primarily recommended for the warm-up or cool-down phases of an aerobic workout. We illustrate and briefly describe each exercise with specific reference to its purpose or objective, rehabilitative benefit(s), starting position, and sequence. In some instances, we suggest special considerations and/or modifications that the creative exercise leader can further adapt. Although selected activities are shown in this chapter, a more complete listing is available elsewhere (17).

The number of repetitions of each activity or the time allotted for the activity is left to the exercise leader's discretion. The axiom to remember is, "Avoid boredom." The exercise leader should frequently change postures, activities, and expectations, making the exercise sessions challenging but enjoyable.

Seated Stretch With Ball

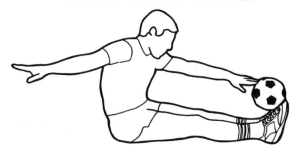

Objective: To stretch the muscles of the lower back and legs

Rehabilitative Benefit: Flexibility

Sequence: Sit, holding a ball on the toes with the fingertips, legs extended or slightly flexed at the knee. Alternate the hand position as shown, maintaining the ball on the instep.

Seated Figure-Eight Ball Movement Under the Legs

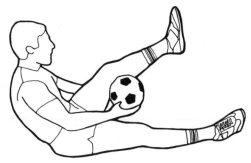

Objective: To stretch the muscles of the lower back and legs

Rehabilitative Benefit: Flexibility, neuromuscular skill

Sequence: Sit, holding a ball, with the legs extended. Alternately raising one leg off the gym floor and then the other, move the ball under the knees from one hand to another.

Caution: Participants should be encouraged to avoid the Valsalva maneuver (breath-holding) during this exercise.

Ball Roll on Floor, Leaning Forward

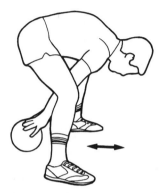

Objective: To stretch the muscles of the lower back, arms, shoulders, and legs

Rehabilitative Benefit: Flexibility

Sequence: Stand, with the feet shoulder-width or further apart, knees slightly flexed, leaning forward at the waist, back gently curved. Roll the ball forward and backward between the feet, attempting to move it at least 6 to 12 inches behind the heels. Keep head up.

Figure-Eight Ball Movement on Gym Floor

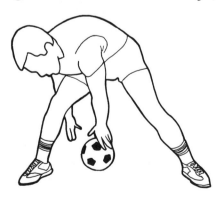

Objective: To stretch the muscles of the lower back, arms, and legs

Rehabilitative Benefits: Flexibility, neuromuscular skill

Sequence: Stand, with the feet wide apart, legs slightly flexed at the knee joint, leaning forward at the waist, focused on the ball. Move the ball on the floor in a figure-eight position, around and between the feet.

Figure-Eight Ball Movement in the Air (off Floor)

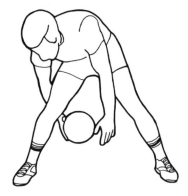

Objective: To stretch the muscles of the lower back, arms, and legs

Rehabilitative Benefits: Flexibility, neuromuscular skill

Sequence: Stand, with feet wide apart, legs slightly flexed at the knee joint, leaning forward at the waist, holding the ball as shown. Move the ball with the hands in a figure-eight position around and between the legs, keeping the ball in the air.

Partner Stationary Activities

The following partner exercises using a playground ball, volleyball, or soccer ball are primarily designed for the warm-up and cool-down components of the exercise session. These activities offer the challenge of working with another person on specific agility and movement skills while simultaneously enhancing balance and flexibility. Some exercises involve precision timing, whereas others require hand-eye coordination.

Selected partner stationary exercises include the following:

Partner Shoulder Stretch With Ball

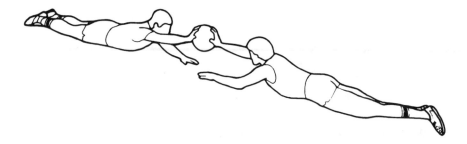

Objective: To stretch the muscles of the arms, shoulders, and lower back

Rehabilitative Benefits: Flexibility, neuromuscular skill

Sequence: Start in the prone position, with one hand on the ground and the other hand holding a ball in midair, 6 to 10 inches above the gym floor. Lower the ball to the ground, change hands, and lift ball again to starting position. Both partners should use the *same* hand, that is, either both right or both left, when holding the ball in mid–air.

Partner Static Stretch With Ball

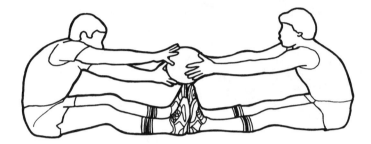

Objective: To stretch the muscles of the arms, shoulders, lower back, and legs

Rehabilitative Benefits: Flexibility

Sequence: Sit, facing a partner, feet against feet, legs flat on the floor or slightly flexed at the knee joint, holding a ball simultaneously over the feet for 5 to 15 seconds. Alternatively, the partners may pass the ball to each other, leaning forward as the ball is exchanged.

Ball Suspension With Partner

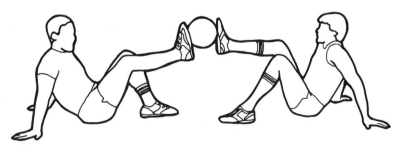

Objective: To stretch and tone the muscles of the abdomen, lower back, and arms

Rehabilitative Benefits: Strength, muscular endurance

Sequence: Sit, facing a partner, hands on floor for support, both legs flexed, with one foot on the floor and the other holding a ball against the partner's outstretched foot. Alternate feet so as to maintain the ball in midair position. Both partners should use the *same* leg, that is, either both right or both left, when supporting the ball in midair.

> **Note:** Ball suspension with partner can be made even more challenging if the exercise leader walks among the pairs of participants, tossing a separate sport ball. The participants catch the ball while maintaining the specified position (i.e., ball in midair, pressed between the feet) and throw it back to the leader.

Seated Ball Foot-Flick With Partner

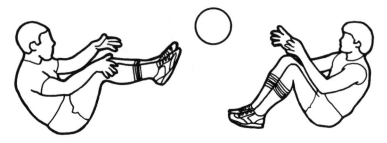

Objective: To stretch and tone the muscles of the abdomen and lower back

Rehabilitative Benefits: Strength, muscular endurance, neuromuscular skill

Sequence: Sit, facing a partner, knees bent, feet together on the floor. One partner places the ball on the knees, letting it roll down the legs toward the feet. At the last second, he/she suddenly raises feet off the floor, flicking the ball to the partner, who catches it and repeats the sequence.

Partner Balance With Ball Exchange

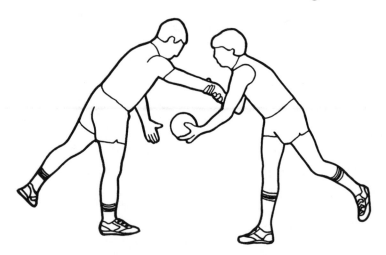

a.

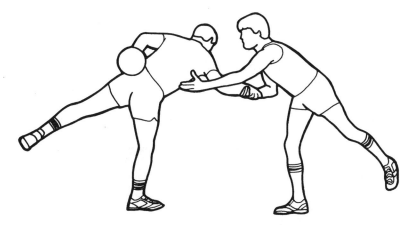

b.

Objective: To enhance balance, flexibility, and coordination

Rehabilitative Benefits: Flexibility, neuromuscular skill

Sequence: Stand, facing partner, lock wrists, and balance on one leg while extending the other leg rearward, in the air. Hand the ball back and forth, under the arm, behind the back, or beneath the support or non–support leg.

Back-to-Back Ball Exchange With Partner

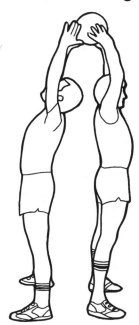

a.

Objective: To stretch the muscles of the lower back, arms, shoulders, and legs

Rehabilitative Benefits: Flexibility

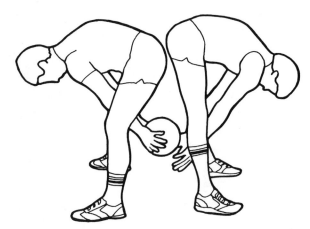

b.

Sequence: Stand, back-to-back, slightly separated, with feet shoulder–width apart. Hand the ball over the head (arms extended) and between the legs as shown. Repeat several times.

Side Twist With Ball Exchange

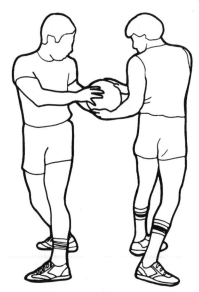

Objective: To stretch the muscles of the back, shoulders, arms, and abdomen

Rehabilitative Benefits: Flexibility

Sequence: Stand, back-to-back, about 2 feet from a partner, knees slightly flexed, feet forward. One partner holds a ball. Both rotate in the same direction (e.g., both to the right) so that the ball can be handed off as shown. The partners now rotate in the opposite direction (e.g., both to the left), and the ball is exchanged again.

Ball Roll to Partner

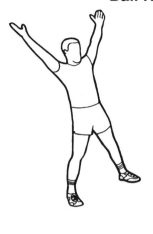

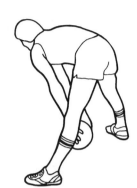

a.

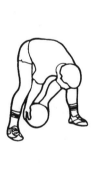

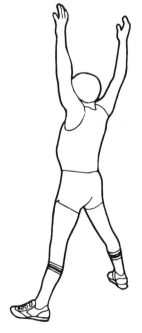

b.

Objective: To stretch the muscles of the arms, legs, lower back, and torso

Rehabilitative Benefits: Flexibility, neuromuscular skill

Sequence: Stand, facing partner, approximately 10 to 15 feet from each other, feet wide apart (i.e., more than shoulder-width). One partner bends forward at the waist and rolls the ball on floor to opposite partner, stretching the arms above the head at the conclusion of the movement. The other partner then repeats the roll, and so on.

Note: This exercise is even more challenging if partners face opposite directions. Since the partners cannot initially see the ball rolling toward them, precise timing is required.

Foot Ball-Tap With Partner

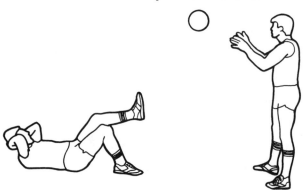

Objective: To stretch and tone the muscles of the legs and abdomen

Rehabilitative Benefits: Flexibility, muscular endurance

Sequence: One person lies on his/her back, supporting the neck with the hands, and places one foot on the ground (knee flexed) while raising the other leg and foot. A partner stands 4 to 6 feet from him, holding a ball. The partner tosses the ball *underhand* toward the raised foot of the person on the ground. The person on the ground taps the ball back to the standing partner, who catches it. The sequence is continued, alternating feet.

Ball Drop, Knee Kick With Partner

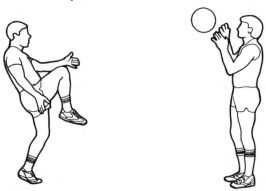

Objective: To stretch and tone the muscles of the legs and abdomen

Rehabilitative Benefits: Flexibility, muscular endurance, neuromuscular skill

Sequence: Stand, facing a partner, about 5 to 10 feet apart, with the other person holding a ball at shoulder height. This person drops the ball and simultaneously raises his/her leg, flexing the knee, so that the ball hits the front portion of the thigh and then bounces to the partner, who catches it and repeats the sequence. Alternate the raised leg with each turn.

Ball Toss With Partner, Balancing on One Leg

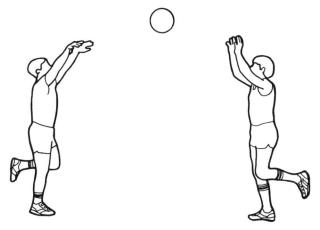

Objective: To enhance balance and agility and gradually raise the heart rate

Rehabilitative Benefits: Neuromuscular skill, strength, muscular endurance

Sequence: Stand, facing a partner while balancing on one leg, one partner holding a ball. Toss the ball back and forth between partners while alternating the support leg with each toss.

Behind-the-Back Ball Toss to Partner

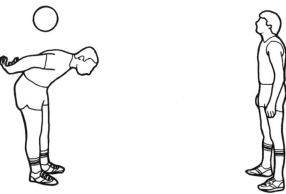

Objective: To stretch the muscles of the arms, shoulders, lower back, and abdomen

Rehabilitative Benefits: Flexibility, neuromuscular skill

Sequence: Stand, facing a partner, about 10 to 15 feet apart, with one person holding a ball behind the back with both hands, arms squeezed tightly against the sides of the ball. The person holding the ball bends forward at the waist, tossing the ball to his partner, who catches it and repeats the movement.

Ball Juggling With Partner

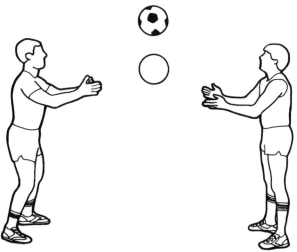

Objective: To promote hand-eye coordination and agility

Rehabilitative Benefits: Neuromuscular skill

Sequence: Stand, about 6 to 15 feet from a partner, with each person holding a ball. Toss balls simultaneously to each other, one person tossing "low" and the other tossing "high," and each person then alternating between low and high. A floor bounce can be included in the sequence.

INDIVIDUAL CONTINUOUS-MOVEMENT ACTIVITIES

The following individual activities, using a playground ball or volleyball, are designed primarily for the cardiorespiratory portion of the warm-up or as a complement to the endurance phase. Ideally, these aerobic activities should follow the musculoskeletal portion of the warm-up (i.e., stretching, flexibility, and muscle-strengthening exercises) and involve an intensity sufficient to evoke a heart rate response within 20 beats/minute of the heart rate prescribed for endurance training.

Here we illustrate selected individual continuous-movement activities.

Foot Dribble Around Gymnasium

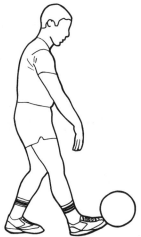

Objective: To improve agility and increase the heart rate

Rehabilitative Benefits: Neuromuscular skill, cardiorespiratory endurance, body composition (trimness)

Sequence: Stand, with the ball on the floor in front of the feet. Tap the ball gently, using either the medial or the lateral portions of the foot or toes, while walking around the perimeter of the gymnasium.

> ***Note:*** Caution the exerciser to avoid tripping on the ball.

Ball Roll Down Back While Walking

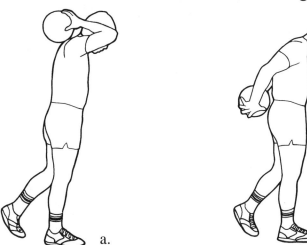

a.   b.

Objective: To stretch the muscles of the arms and shoulders while gradually raising the heart rate

Rehabilitative Benefits: Flexibility, neuromuscular skill, cardiorespiratory endurance, body composition (trimness)

Sequence: Stand, holding a ball on the upper back between the shoulder blades. Then walk, gently leaning forward and curving the back, releasing the ball. Quickly move both hands to the position shown, so as to catch the ball at the lower back (before it drops to the ground). Repeat.

Overhead Ball Stretch While Walking

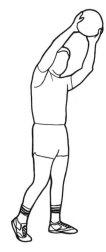

Objective: To stretch the muscles of the upper extremities and torso and gradually raise the heart rate

Rehabilitative Benefits: Flexibility, cardiorespiratory endurance, body composition (trimness)

Sequence: Stand, arms outstretched to hold a ball over the head. While maintaining this position, walk briskly, gently bending the trunk from side to side.

Ball Toss Against Wall While Sidestepping

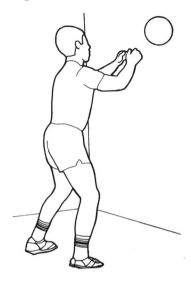

Objective: To promote agility and gradually increase the heart rate

Rehabilitative Benefits: Neuromuscular skill, cardiorespiratory endurance, body composition (trimness)

Sequence: Stand, facing a wall, feet apart, while holding a ball. Sidestepping around the perimeter of the gymnasium, toss the ball against the walls and catch it.

PARTNER CONTINUOUS-MOVEMENT ACTIVITIES

The following partner activities, involving a playground ball or volleyball, can be used for the cardiorespiratory portion of the warm-up or to complement the endurance phase. However, with partner continuous–movement activities, participants should be paired with individuals who have similar aerobic fitness levels. The number of repetitions of each activity or time allotted for them is left to the exercise leader's discretion.

Selected partner continuous-movement activities include the following.

Ball Arch With Partner While Walking

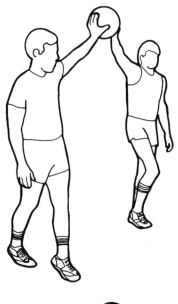

a.

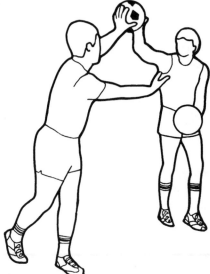

b.

Objective: To stretch the arm and shoulder muscles and gradually raise the heart rate

Rehabilitative Benefits: Flexibility, cardiorespiratory endurance, body composition (trimness)

Sequence: Walk, side by side with a partner, with a ball held overhead as illustrated. As a modification of this activity, another ball can be tossed with the outside arm from one partner to the other.

Ball Toss With Partner While Sidestepping

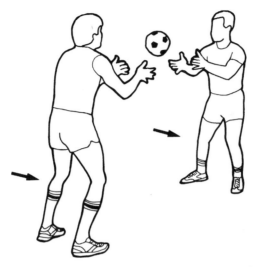

Objective: To promote lateral agility and gradually raise the heart rate

Rehabilitative Benefits: Neuromuscular skill, cardiorespiratory endurance, body composition (trimness)

Sequence: Stand, facing a partner, about 4 to 6 feet apart, with one partner holding a ball. While slowly sidestepping across the floor, the partners toss the ball back and forth to each other.

Ball-on-Back Agility Drill With Partner

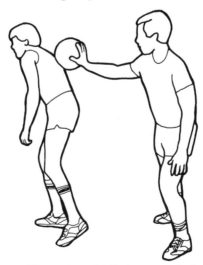

Objective: To promote agility and gradually increase the heart rate

Rehabilitative Benefits: Neuromuscular skill, cardiorespiratory endurance, body composition (trimness)

Sequence: Place the ball on the partner's back, between the shoulder blades, with one hand. The partner with the ball on his/her back begins *walking slowly,* changing directions frequently, to cause the other person to lose control of the ball.

Ball Toss With Partner, Alternating Positions

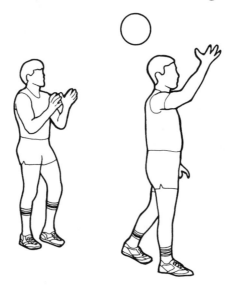

Objective: To stretch the arm and shoulder muscles and gradually raise the heart rate

Rehabilitative Benefits: Flexibility, neuromuscular skill, cardiorespiratory endurance, body composition (trimness)

Sequence: Stand, one partner in front of the other, with the front partner holding a ball. Both individuals start walking, and the front partner tosses the ball over his/her shoulder to the back partner, who catches it. The back partner now walks briskly ahead, changing positions, and the sequence is repeated.

GROUP ACTIVITIES

The following activities, using a playground ball or volleyball, are designed mainly to complement the warm-up, cool-down, and endurance components of the exercise session. *Note: Although only two persons are shown in each of the illustrations, group activities generally involve 6 to 20 or more participants.* The number of repetitions of each activity and the time allotted for them are left to the exercise leader's discretion.

In the following we illustrate selected group activities.

Ball Roll With Participants Sitting in a Circle

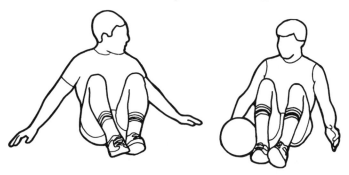

Objective: To tone and strengthen the abdominal muscles—and have fun

Rehabilitative Benefits: Muscular endurance, strength, flexibility

Sequence: This activity requires several exercisers who are sitting in a circle, facing inward. The ball is rolled on the floor, to the right or to the left, under the participants' legs. The feet should be raised off the floor, knees together, as the ball goes under the legs.

Ball Passing (With Feet) Around Circle

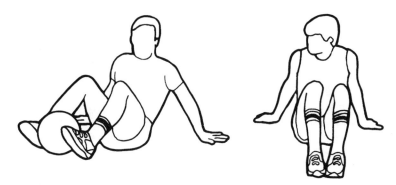

Objective: To tone and strengthen the abdominal muscles

Rehabilitative Benefits: Strength, muscular endurance, neuromuscular skill

Sequence: This exercise requires several participants who are sitting in a circle, facing inward. As the ball is lifted with the feet, the participant rotates on his/her "seat" and places the ball on the gym floor to the person next to him, who continues the sequence.

> **Note:** Participants should be cautioned to avoid breath-holding during this activity. The ball should *not* be passed in mid–air from one participant to another.

Back-of-the-Hand Ball Balance While Walking

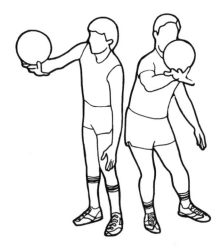

Objective: To promote agility and coordination and gradually raise the heart rate

Rehabilitative Benefits: Neuromuscular skill, cardiorespiratory endurance, body composition (trimness)

Sequence: On a large gym floor and with a number of participants (i.e., 6 to 20), each person balances a playground ball on the *back* of the hand (fingers and arm outstretched), palm facing the floor, as shown. Participants begin walking in different directions while keeping the ball balanced on the back of the hand. If the ball drops to the floor, or if the opposite hand or the chest is used to stabilize the ball, the participant is "out." Nevertheless, those who are "out" should continue walking and/or dribbling the ball around the perimeter of the gymnasium. The last participant to have the ball in position is the "winner."

> **Note:** This activity can be made even more challenging (and fun) by encouraging participants to "gently bump" hips as they walk past each other in an attempt to make someone else lose control of his/her ball.

GAMES AND RELAYS

Participants in an exercise-based rehabilitation program have a medically defined cardiovascular condition, often with accompanying functional limitations. They have been informed that physical activity in the appropriate dosage and frequency will result in positive physiological changes. What they haven't been told is that this shared experience with others can be an enjoyable one. Programs that offer the same old stuff (SOS) three times weekly, session after session, are boring to the participant and of little challenge to the exercise leader. One technique that is guaranteed to stimulate enthusiasm among participants is the playing of games and relays. Social interaction is enhanced by these activities, which add an element of camaraderie to the group.

Games and relays lend a pleasurable dimension to an exercise session. Participants perceive this component of the program as a reward for successfully completing the aerobic or stimulus phase of conditioning. Play is the essential element of games. By definition, play is self-expression for the sake of self-expression. The participant has fun. Education of the participants by the exercise leader is critical to the success of playing games. Conventional attitudes toward winning, officiating, game rules, and number of team members, for example, require modification.

In the traditional approach to games and relays, there is a winner and a loser. This aspect of competition is not necessary in cardiac rehabilitation programs. There is no justification for a game to elevate heart rates beyond acceptable targets or for permitting participants' emotions (e.g., desire to win) to become disruptive to themselves or to the group.

Games and relays are played with a purpose. Developing cardiovascular endurance is not the primary goal, as it is during the aerobic phase of the exercise session. Motor skills of agility, balance, and flexibility are the key components of most games and relays. Emphasis should be placed on refining neuromuscular skills and reviving those basic motor skills that in all likelihood have regressed over the years. There is also a therapeutic purpose. Adults are often characterized by a laxity of the abdominal muscles and foreshortening of flexor muscles of the arms and legs. Standing posture tends to be slumped. In the selection of games and relays, attention is given to simple rhythmic movements performed at a moderate pace with emphasis on an extended range of motion. In order to ensure safe performance of games and relays, the exercise leader's responsibility entails following well-defined guidelines.

Selecting appropriate games calls for making objective decisions. An exercise leader must select games based on the participants' ages, gender, and aerobic capacity; on individual skill levels; and on the space available. Choosing games based on age and gender should be viewed as a challenge and not as a problem. Fitness instructors should have a perception of participants' comfort with incidental contact with others as well as their willingness to try various forms of physical activity. Select activities carefully to avoid personal embarrassment. An elementary children's game, for example, may be inappropriate for men and women 40 to 65 years of age.

Individual skill level is often diverse in adult fitness and exercise-based rehabilitation programs. There are participants with superb neuromuscular skills and there are others, who constitute the majority, who are less gifted. Therefore, activities that emphasize large–muscle action or basic motor skills are essential. Keeping the skills required to a minimum permits a continuity of play and a feeling of success. With slight modifications, any game can be altered to meet space and group needs. Road cones are excellent boundary–line markers. Innovation is a key requisite to the success of the game played.

Games selected should be those that are physiologically, anatomically, and kinesiologically sound. Any game activity must permit the leader to control the intensity. For example, soccer, which has a large anaerobic component, would be an inappropriate activity for a post-myocardial infarction, phase III participant. However, if only fast walking is permitted, the intensity is reduced dramatically. Walking speeds of 4 mph require a 4+ MET energy expenditure, which is safely within the tolerance of a participant who has a 5 to 6 MET exercise–training intensity. Monitoring heart rate for 10 seconds is a useful technique for periodically decreasing the intensity of play. Additional modifications could include requiring participants to foot-check or stop the ball before foot-passing it to a team member. Other rules could stipulate that the participant on offense has the "right-of-way" and that only one foot dribble is permitted before the ball is passed. A leader can control the intensity of the activity. Safety of the game player is paramount.

A kinesiologically sound activity is one that is within the repertoire of motor skills of the participant. To use soccer again as an example, an exercise leader should never introduce a game until the participants feel comfortable with ball–dribbling and ball-passing skills. These skills can be practiced at any age. A few minutes of the time allotted for games can be devoted to skill development. Sport balls can be used in warm-up activity or during a stimulus or aerobic phase. Use of a volleyball or sport ball that is lighter in weight is preferable to the use of a soccer ball, which is heavier.

The nomenclature or terminology used to describe movement or formations requires educating the participant. Using the correct terminology saves time and words and is necessary to move participants about a space rapidly. Many mass activities use geometric formations, such as a square, circle, rectangle, triangle, or a U. For example, a starting formation for a game may be a circle of 8 participants, or a double circle in which 8 participants in the outside ring face inward and 8 participants in the inner ring face outward. The vocabulary used is a verbal shorthand. For relays, the file and the flank rank are two common formations. A leader would ask a group of 12 participants to line up in two files of 6. This would mean that each participant faces the back of the person directly in front of him or her. Or the command could be two flank ranks of 6. Participants would line up shoulder to shoulder facing forward. Although there is some leadership autocracy in the technique, it accomplishes the task of moving a number of participants safely and efficiently. To complement the terminology for formation, one should educate participants on the movement of the body and its extremities. Commands are given for actual movements. For example, "Raise your right arm to full extension," "Lower your upper body to hip height," "Flex your legs at the knee joint," and so on. Being precise leaves little room for misinterpretation. When precision is coupled with a visual demonstration, participants quickly learn what is expected of them.

Reducing the participant's risk of injury is a challenge to the exercise leader. There should be sufficient space and planning to permit games to be played without collision with objects, walls, equipment, and other participants. When two or more groups are active, overlapping boundary lines of courts should be avoided. Another safety issue that requires attention is the playing surface. Slippery surfaces are contraindicated. Finally, the games selected should avoid sudden twisting and turning of the body, and special consideration should be given to the lower extremities.

The exercise leader should use sound elementary pedagogical techniques. For outdoor activities, these would include having the participants' backs to the sun and wind when talking to them. Modulating the voice and speaking clearly are important communication skills. Any game played should have few rules, but these must be enforced; for example, when a participant inappropriately runs during a walking game, it is considered an infraction and the violation results in a point for the opposing side, a side out, or return of the ball to the spot of the infraction.

Directions for movement patterns must be clearly explained to participants—for example, in relay types of games, "Walk to the right," "Move in a clockwise direction." The participants should walk through the activity—first as a warm-up and second as rehearsal to the activity itself.

Sight and hearing acuity of older adults is also a concern. When participants are wearing corrective eyeglasses, they should wear protective glass guards similar to those worn by racquetball or squash racquet players. Several additional pairs of eye guards should be in the inventory of equipment and should be available for use by participants when sport ball activities will be part of games and relays.

Acoustics in larger rooms or gymnasiums are often a problem. In these settings, even persons without sound deficiencies may not hear the instructions or commands of the exercise leader. Therefore, in addition to a controlled inflected voice, the leader should use hand and arm signals to complement the verbal instructions. Eye contact and maintaining the attention of the participants are also important.

Since activity is the primary concern, involve all participants and avoid elimination-type games. It's not fun (or effective) for people to be left out of group play. When games appear to be at the height of enthusiasm, stop them and move rapidly to another activity. This technique will decrease the intensity of the activity, and participants will look forward to playing the game on another occasion.

Two issues seldom addressed in exercise programs for the older man or woman are balance and the fear of falling. Balance may be affected by medical problems—diabetes, for example—or medications. However, the majority of adults lack static or dynamic balance abilities because the skills are seldom rehearsed or practiced. Balance activity can be incorporated into relays or practiced individually with a sport ball. The "stork stand," with the sole of the foot in contact with the medial aspect of the knee joint of the support leg, and hands on hips, is a good introductory skill. Alternating support legs, after a 10-15-second wait, adds a dynamic component. Using a sport ball, the participant can circle it about the waist or the single support leg, or toss it from hand to hand. The variations are limitless.

Fear of falling is a concern because falling is never practiced. It is a catastrophic event that often results in a fracture. A common one is the Colles fracture—the fracture of the lower end of the radius with the lower bone fragment displaced posteriorly. Why? Because in a backward fall, the arm is extended and the hand is rotated to break the fall. The torque and body weight result in an anatomical overload, and a fracture results.

But falling forward and backward can be practiced. Using mats and assuming a front support position, participants can safely perform left and right shoulder rolls. They should do these movements slowly and with leader instruction and support. Fear of falling can be overcome with practice.

An exercise leader should have an extensive knowledge inventory of games and relays. However, the group will have favorite activities. Use these activities sparingly. They are to be enjoyed, but not overdone.

Introducing new games and relays should be an ongoing process. However, they may not all be well received. For a variety of reasons, there are "duds." The motor coordination skills required may be overly complex, or the game itself may be too complicated for the participants to quickly grasp. This does not mean that when introduced to another group at another time the activity will not be successful. When you recognize that participant interest has waned, stop the activity and move to another.

Incorporating games and relays into an exercise-based rehabilitation program should be a challenge to the fitness instructor as well as the participant. Exercise is a science. Leading physical activity is an art form. Success of the games component rests with the leader's ability to be creative, imaginative, and flexible.

Games

Bounce Ball

Rehabilitative Benefit: Neuromuscular skill

The Field: Any open playing area; no boundaries are necessary. The equivalent of a net divides the area into two equal sections: the "net" consists of a line drawn on the court, a rope set at a height not exceeding knee height, or an obstacle such as a player's bench.

Players: Equal number on each team; the smaller the area, the fewer the players

Playing Time: Some length of time that is acceptable to both teams

Equipment: Some light bounce ball, sport ball, volleyball or European handball

The Game: The game starts when a player strikes the ball with the palm of her hand, a closed fist, or the back of her hand. The ball must land on the ground on the player's own side of the "net" and then bounce over the "net." The opponents then return the ball over the "net" after the ball has hit the ground on their side of the "net." The ball may be passed from team member to team member (as in volleyball) for a maximum of three times before it must be directed over the "net" after hitting the ground. The ball may hit the ground once or not at all when being passed from one team member to another. The basic rule is that the ball must be bounced off the floor before going over the "net."

Scoring: The serving team scores one point for every time the opponents fail to return the ball correctly. If the serving team fails to direct the ball across the "net," the opponents score one point and are given the serve. The serve changes every time the non–serving team becomes the serving team. Players rotate so that each player has an opportunity to serve.

Modified German Handball or 3-3-3

Rehabilitative Benefit: Neuromuscular skill, cardiorespiratory endurance

The Field: Any open playing area, field, or gymnasium with a goal at each end; goal size 3-4 yards

Players: Equal numbers on each team; the smaller the area, the fewer the players

Playing Time: Some length of time acceptable to both teams

Equipment: A European handball

The Game: The game begins with a throw from the throwing team's goal line. The ball must not touch the ground; if it does, the ball is immediately, with no delay of game, taken by the team that did not touch the ball. An interception that is dropped to the ground is then given to the team that threw the ball. A successful interception gives the ball to the intercepting team. A ball that has been caught by a member of the throwing team (or intercepting team) may then be (1) held for up to 3 seconds, then thrown to a team member; (2) moved forward three paces before being thrown again; or (3) thrown immediately to a team member. In this manner, the ball is moved to the opponent's goal line; here it must be thrown through the goal after having hit the ground one or more times. (This is the only time the ball may hit the ground.) The winner is the team with the most goals. If the ball goes out of bounds, it is given to the opponent, who will restart the game with a throw from where the ball went out of bounds.

Penalties: A no-contact game. A penalty is charged against the team causing contact: this is simply a free throw into the field of play.

Soccer

Rehabilitative Benefit: Neuromuscular skill, cardiorespiratory endurance, body composition (trimness)

The Field: Any open playing area, field, or gymnasium with a goal at each end; goal size 3-4 yards

Standards: Pylons or cages may be used

Players: Equal number on each team

Playing Time: Length of time acceptable to exercise leader

Equipment: Any type of sport ball

The Game: The game is started by having one side advance the soccer ball, using the foot, toward the opponent's goal. No body contact is permitted. The game is one of walking, striding, or jogging. Running is a violation. The ball may be intercepted. Goalies are frequently changed. No location is out-of-bounds in a gymnasium, as the walls may be used to facilitate foot passing from one player to another. The winner is the team with the most goals.

Penalties: A no-contact game. Penalty is charged against the team causing contact; the opposing team receives the ball to put it back in play.

Modified Volleyball or Bounce Volleyball

Rehabilitative Benefit: Neuromuscular skill

The Field: Volleyball court with a net height not to exceed 8 feet. Any height between 5 and 8 feet is acceptable. A rope may be used if a net is not available. When a large gymnasium space is available, the standard court, 30 by 60, is ignored and the entire gymnasium may be in play. When teams have a player advantage, the exercise leader should rotate players to the opposing side so that participants have equal opportunity to play.

Players: Any number may play; with larger groups, two courts may be used.

Playing Time: Length of time acceptable to the exercise leader

Equipment: Volleyball

The Game: The game is started when a player strikes the ball over the net. It may be returned by the opponent in a wide variety of ways. It may be struck sharply or hit underhand or overhand; or if the opponent is not able to strike the ball in flight, a floor bounce is permitted (bounce volleyball). Generally, at least one and no more than three bounces are permitted on the return side (i.e., after the serve). This is determined *before* play starts. There is, however, no limit on how many players may strike the ball (as opposed to bouncing it) before getting it back over the net. A point is scored when one team returns the ball over the net successfully one more time than the opponent.

Penalties: Side out is declared when the ball is struck more than one time in succession by a single player.

Kickball Golf (Out-of-Doors Activity)

Rehabilitative Benefit: Neuromuscular skill, cardiorespiratory endurance, body composition (trimness)

The Field: Any outside area that includes trees, telephone poles, or implanted poles. The game should be played in a relatively open area, approximately 80-200 yards.

Players: Any number of participants can be involved. Play may be individual, paired, or team.

Playing Time: The length of time acceptable to the exercise leader

Equipment: A wide variety of sport balls to include volleyball, soccer ball, and balls of various circumferences

The Game: An arbitrary tee is established by the exercise leader, who creates his own golf hole. Before the players tee off, the leader determines the par for the hole by evaluating the distance, hazards, and terrain (e.g., downsloping) that may be encountered. For example, a hole that is 180 yards might be considered a Par 5 while a 60-yard hole might be a Par 3. Participants must walk briskly or jog slowly between kicks. The ball is drop-kicked, punted, or kicked from the ground. The participant's best kicking skill is employed. The object of the game is to strike the pin (flag) in the fewest number of strokes. The basic rule is to continue movement.

Scoring: The success of the game is dependent upon the leader's ability to create a golf course that is interesting and challenging. Many variations are possible, such as kicking the ball with the nondominant foot, the presence of doglegs, or obstacles that may be in the path of the kickball golfer. The least number of kicks on a predetermined number of holes determines the champion. For a variation, the exercise leader may select a participant to identify the next hole and give the prescribed number of kicks required for par.

Comment: The activity is not a primary means of conditioning, but it complements the aerobic conditioning program, sustains attention, and provides an element of fun.

Relays

Figure Eights

Rehabilitative Benefit: Neuromuscular skill

Starting Formation: File; sitting, standing, or kneeling

Players: Equal numbers in two, three, or four files

Playing Time: All participants should have at least one turn at going from the rear to the front of the file.

Equipment: Medicine ball, soccer ball, or volleyball

The Relay: While seated, the person at the head of the file passes a sport ball overhead to the person directly behind. The last person walks rapidly or jogs in a figure-eight pattern between other players and begins the sequence again by passing the sport ball overhead.

Variations:

1. Foot dribbling of the ball.
2. In a standing position, the first person passes the ball overhead, the second person passes the ball between his/her legs, and so on.
3. In a standing position, the first person rotates 180° to the right and hands off the ball, the second person rotates 180° to the left, etc.
4. Similar activities from a kneeling position if out-of-doors.

Clock Relay

Rehabilitative Benefit: Neuromuscular skill

Starting Formation: Two or more circles with participants lying in the prone position, facing inward.

Players: Equal numbers in each circle, generally six, seven, or eight.

Playing Time: All participants should have at least one turn.

Equipment: Sport balls can be used.

The Relay: One player on command moves from a front–lying to a standing position and walks rapidly or jogs in a clockwise direction. As he passes over the first person, that player moves from the front–lying position to the standing position and follows the leader over the second person. On completing the 360° circle, the leader assumes the front-lying position as remaining team members complete their turns.

Recommendation: Walk through the relay one time.

Variations:
1. Each participant has a sport ball and air dribbles the ball while completing the 360° circle. Ball dribbling can also be performed.
2. Rather than walking or jogging, the player can skip or hop.

Shuttle Relay

Rehabilitative Benefit: Neuromuscular skill

Starting Formation: Two or more files with half of the players 15 to 20 feet from their team members, who face them in their file formation. Starting position: standing or seated.

Players: Equal numbers, 6-10 participants per shuttle

Playing Time: Continuous movement for 2 to 5 minutes in duration

Equipment: Sport ball to include medicine balls, soccer balls, volleyballs, mush or fleece balls

The Relay: Continuous movement; the first person in the file walks or jogs the distance between the team file and either hands off to, tosses a ball to, or touches his teammate and proceeds to the right of the file formation to become the last person in the file. The player touched or receiving the ball moves the distance between file play members and touches or hands off the ball to the team player to his immediate front. The relay involves continuous movement until all participants have had at least one turn.

Variations:
1. Foot dribbling or hand dribbling a sport ball.

2. Air dribbling while foot dribbling a second ball.
3. Rope skipping.
4. Bounce–passing or overhead passing of a basketball.

Conclusion

Adult fitness and exercise-based cardiac rehabilitation programs should be safe, effective, and enjoyable. Moreover, exercise leaders should educate and motivate participants. The principles, ideas, and activities described in this chapter can help you to achieve these objectives. We have used them over the years with good adherence in our programs. You can also use these program suggestions and aerobic activities, or modifications of them, with children, senior citizens, or people who use a wheelchair—and in the exercise programming of a broad spectrum of patients, including those with intermittent claudication, obesity, diabetes, osteoporosis, and chronic obstructive pulmonary disease.

One advantage of the "Games-As-Aerobics" approach is that it maximizes group support and camaraderie by using sports equipment (e.g., playground balls) in creative activities, games, or relays that emphasize cooperation (rather than competition), fun, variety, and success. Exercise leaders should select those activities that are best suited to the cardiovascular and musculoskeletal conditions of their participants, and adapt or modify others—yielding literally thousands of variations to the themes that have been presented.

The challenge is yours!

References

1. McDonough, J.R., Kusumi, F., and Bruce, R.A. Variations in maximal oxygen intake with physical activity in middle-aged men. *Circulation,* **41**, 743-751; 1970.
2. Franklin, B.A. How much exercise is enough? *Encyclopedia Britannica, Medical and Health Annual* (pp. 471-476); 1993.
3. Ornish, D.M., Scherwitz, L.W., Doody, R.S., et al. Effects of stress management training and dietary changes in treating ischemic heart disease. *Journal of the American Medical Association,* **249**, 54-59; 1983.
4. Wenger, N.K., Froelicher, E.S., Smith, L.K., et al. *Cardiac rehabilitation as secondary prevention. Clinical practice guideline. Quick reference guide for clinicians,* No. 17 (AHCPR Publication No. 96-0673). Rockville, MD: U.S. Department of Health and Human Services, Public Health Service, Agency for Health Care Policy and Research and National Heart, Lung, and Blood Institute; October 1995.
5. Franklin, B.A. Program factors that influence exercise adherence: Practical adherence skills for the clinical staff. In R. Dishman (Ed.), *Exercise adherence: Its impact on public health* (pp. 237-258). Champaign, IL: Human Kinetics; 1988.

6. Rejeski, W.J., and Kenney, E.A. *Fitness motivation: preventing participant dropout.* Champaign, IL: Life Enhancement; 1988.

7. Oldridge, N.B. Adherence to adult exercise fitness programs. In J.D. Matarazzo, S.M. Weiss, J.A. Herd, and N.E. Miller (Eds.), *Behavioral health: A handbook of health enhancement and disease prevention* (pp. 467-487). New York: Wiley; 1984.

8. Annesi, J.J. *Enhancing exercise motivation: A guide to increasing fitness center member retention.* Los Angeles: Leisure; 1996.

9. Perry, P. Are we having fun yet? *American Health Magazine* pp. 59-63; March 1987.

10. Fitness programs held beneficial. *Medical Tribune* pp. 29; March 1965.

11. Massie, J.F., and Shephard, R.J. Physiological and psychological effects of training—a comparison of individual and gymnasium programs, with a characterization of the exercise "drop out." *Medicine and Science in Sports,* **3**:110-117; 1971.

12. Shaw, L.W., et al. Effects of a prescribed supervised exercise program on mortality and cardiovascular morbidity in patients after a myocardial infarction. *American Journal of Cardiology,* **48**, 39-46; 1981.

13. Wilhelmsen, L., Sanne, H., Elmfeldt, D., et al. A controlled trial of physical training after myocardial infarction: Effects on risk factors, nonfatal reinfarction, and death. *Preventive Medicine,* **4**, 491-508; 1975.

14. DeBusk, R.F., Haskell, W.L., Miller, N.H., et al. Medically directed at home rehabilitation soon after clinically uncomplicated myocardial infarction: A new model for patient care. *American Journal of Cardiology,* **55**, 251-257; 1985.

15. Stoedefalke, K.G. Physical fitness programs for adults. *American Journal of Cardiology,* **33**, 787-790; 1974.

16. Stoedefalke, K.G., and Hodgson, J.L. Exercise Rx—designing a program. *Medical Opinion,* **4**, 48-55; 1975.

17. Franklin, B.A., Oldridge, N.B., Stoedefalke, K.G., and Loechel, W.E. *On the ball: innovative activities for adult fitness and cardiac rehabilitation programs.* Carmel, IN: Benchmark Press; 1990.

Index

About the Authors

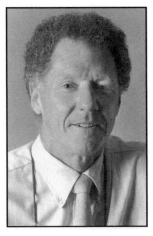

Paul Fardy is a professor in the Department of Family, Nutrition, and Exercise Sciences and the director of Physical Activity and Teenage Health (PATH) at Queens College. A pioneer in developing comprehensive hospital-based programs, Dr. Fardy participated in the National Exercise and Heart Disease Project (NEHDP), a major research trial in cardiac rehabilitation, and has authored or edited six books and more than 100 publications primarily on cardiac rehabilitation and health promotion. In 1996 he received the Outstanding Alumni Award from the State University of New York, the Outstanding Research Award from the New York chapter of the American College of Sports Medicine (ACSM), and the Health Education award for excellence in progamming health education from the New York State Health Department. His program (PATH) was also awarded the 1995 National Award from ACSM for promoting Healthy People 2000 objectives. Dr. Fardy lives in Point Lookout, New York, where he enjoys jogging, biking, beach volleyball, and classical music.

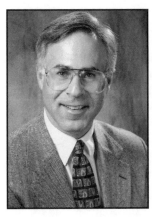

Barry Franklin's credentials include past positions as president of AACVPR, vice president of ACSM, and editor-in-chief of the *Journal of Cardiopulmonary Rehabilitation.* A recipient of AACVPR's Distinguished Service Award and Award of Excellence and the San Diego County Medical Society's Media Award, he's written, edited, or contributed to more than 200 publications on exercise testing and cardiac rehabilitation, including AACVPR's *Guidelines for Cardiovascular Rehabilitation Programs* and the recent *Clinical Practice Guideline on Cardiac Rehabilitation* sponsored by the U.S. Department of Health and Human Services and the Agency for Health Care Policy and Research, National Heart, Lung, and Blood Institute. Dr. Franklin is currently director of the cardiac rehabilitation program and exercise laboratories at William Beaumont Hospital and a professor of physiology at Wayne State University School of Medicine in Detroit. He and his wife, Linda, reside in West Bloomfield, Michigan. His leisure-time activities include golf and distance walking.

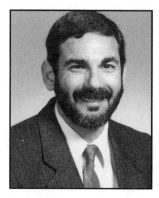

A member of AACVPR's board of directors, **John Porcari** is executive director of the oldest university-based—and possibly the best known—cardiac rehabilitation program in the United States: LaCrosse Exercise and Health Program. He is also a professor in the Exercise and Sports Science Department at the University of Wisconsin La Crosse and teaches an Adult Fitness/Cardiac Rehabilitation graduate program. Dr. Porcari organizes five cardiac rehabilitation, exercise physiology, and pulmonary rehabilitation workshops annually. He has received more than 40 exercise-related research grants, and in 1995 he received the Distinguished Service Award from AACVPR. An avid hunter and recreational fisherman, Dr. Porcari lives in LaCrosse, Wisconsin, with his wife, Marggi, and their two children.

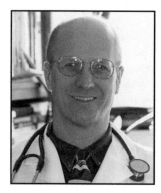

David Verrill is the director of the cardiovascular testing laboratory for Mid Carolina Cardiology and helps to administer cardiac resistive training for the 300 patients of the Mecklenburg Cardiac Rehabilitation Program. In 1996, he coauthored an article published in *Sports Medicine* that received wide acclaim as the most comprehensive research-based article on cardiac weight training to date. Mr. Verrill has presented at state and national conventions, and in 1996 he was named a Fellow of the AACVPR. He has published position papers on body composition assessment and patient monitoring for the North Carolina Cardiopulmonary Rehabilitation Association (NCCRA) and has chaired both the publications and exercise science committees for that state. The NCCRA has awarded him both the Distinguished Service Award and the Award of Excellence. Mr. Verrill, who enjoys basketball, running, skiing, and gardening, and his wife, Susanne, make their home in Matthews, North Carolina.

All four authors are members of AACVPR and ACSM.

Co-authors for Chapters 3 were **Bo Fernhall**, PhD, The George Washington University, Washington D.C., Department of Exercise Science and Tourism Studies; and Philip K. Wilson, EdD, University of Wisconsin La Crosse, Department of Exercise and Sports Science.

Co-author for Chapter 4 was **Karl G. Stoedefalke**, PhD, Professor emeritus, Department of Exercise Science, Penn State University.

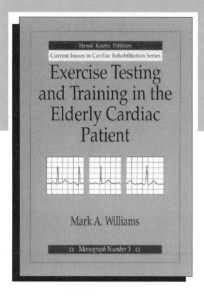
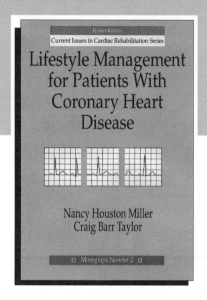